DEDICATED LIVES
Talks with Those Helping Others

Also by Michael Scofield from Sunstone Press

Acting Badly
Making Crazy
Smut Busters
Whirling Backward Into the World
Circus Americana and Other Poems
Sand and Other Flash Fiction

DEDICATED
LIVES

Talks with Those
Helping Others

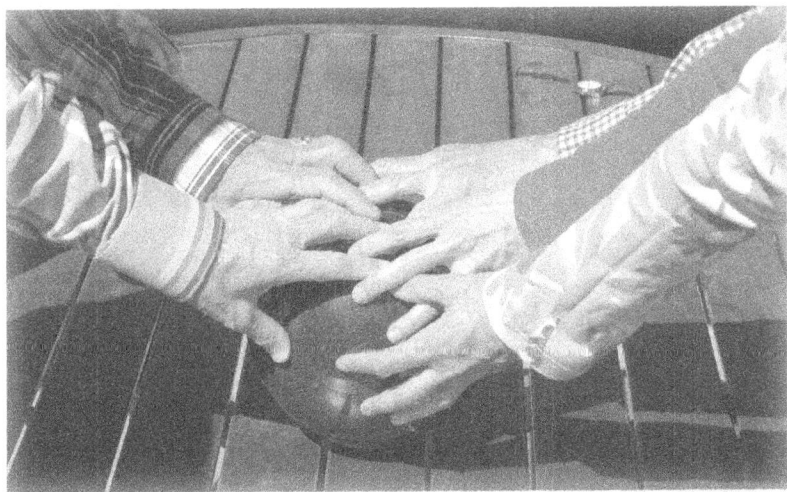

Michael Scofield

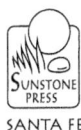

SUNSTONE
PRESS

SANTA FE

Sunstone books may be purchased for educational, business, or sales promotional use.
For information please write: Special Markets Department, Sunstone Press,
P.O. Box 2321, Santa Fe, New Mexico 87504-2321.

Book and cover design › Vicki Ahl
Body typeface › Adobe Caslon Pro
Printed on acid-free paper
∞
eBook 978-1-61139-482-5

Library of Congress Cataloging-in-Publication Data

Names: Scofield, Michael, author.
Title: Dedicated lives : talks with those helping others / by Michael
    Scofield.
Description: Santa Fe : Sunstone Press, [2016]
Identifiers: LCCN 2016026531 (print) | LCCN 2016040657 (ebook) | ISBN
    9781632931375 (softcover : alk. paper) | ISBN 9781611394825
Subjects: LCSH: Social service--United States--Case studies. |
    Humanitarianism--United States--Case studies. | Voluntarism--United
    States--Case studies.
Classification: LCC HV27 .S386 2016 (print) | LCC HV27 (ebook) | DDC
    361.7/40922789--dc23
LC record available at https://lccn.loc.gov/2016026531

SUNSTONE PRESS IS COMMITTED TO MINIMIZING OUR ENVIRONMENTAL IMPACT ON THE PLANET. THE PAPER USED IN THIS BOOK IS FROM RESPONSIBLY MANAGED FORESTS. OUR PRINTER HAS RECEIVED CHAIN OF CUSTODY (COC) CERTIFICATION FROM: THE FOREST STEWARDSHIP COUNCIL™ (FSC®), PROGRAMME FOR THE ENDORSEMENT OF FOREST CERTIFICATION™ (PEFC™), AND THE SUSTAINABLE FORESTRY INITIATIVE® (SFI®). THE FSC® COUNCIL IS A NON-PROFIT ORGANIZATION, PROMOTING THE ENVIRONMENTALLY APPROPRIATE, SOCIALLY BENEFICIAL AND ECONOMICALLY VIABLE MANAGEMENT OF THE WORLD'S FORESTS. FSC® CERTIFICATION IS RECOGNIZED INTERNATIONALLY AS A RIGOROUS ENVIRONMENTAL AND SOCIAL STANDARD FOR RESPONSIBLE FOREST MANAGEMENT.

WWW.SUNSTONEPRESS.COM
SUNSTONE PRESS / POST OFFICE BOX 2321 / SANTA FE, NM 87504-2321 /USA
(505) 988-4418 / ORDERS ONLY (800) 243-5644 / FAX (505) 988-1025

FOR NOREEN

Acknowledgments

So much gratitude to Hannah Kaiser, Larry Lazarus, Matt Roybal, and Marian Shirin for steering me to likely Good Samaritans to interview. Equal gratitude to Sunstone's publisher, Jim Smith, and his assistant, Carl Condit, for their useful advice. Thanks to Vicki Ahl at Sunstone for book design and to Russ Stolins for formatting expertise. Special thanks for copyediting to my late wife, Noreen, as well as to dear friends Irene Webb and Megan Siegel. All information in this book was correct at the time of publication. That includes phone numbers and websites, thanks to Megan Siegel.

Those hands and arms you see on the cover belong to interviewees Jane Clarke, Larry Lazarus, Barbara Rockman, Kim Straus, and the author. Thank you all.

Contents

PREFACE

This book honors the legions of people in this country who are dedicating their lives to helping others. The representative thirteen in-depth talks with fourteen people you're about to eavesdrop on took place from 2014 into 2016, in Santa Fe, New Mexico.

These credits to the human race often involve their families in their work, and borrow evening and weekend hours to get it done. But as Annabelle Montoya, who tells us in the book's second chapter about her work with Alzheimer's patients and their caregivers, explains, "I've always had a passion to help others. It's when I'm happiest. As Mama said, 'Choo Choo, you will never lack for anything because you're always giving.'"

Later, Tony McCarty, who heads up Kitchen Angels, adds, "I guess I'm a little insane because still, after twenty-two years, every time I arrive at one of our events, I love being there, knowing how many of our home-bound clients depend on us for survival."

In these pages you'll get to know a memory-care specialist, a philanthropist, a teacher of poetry, executive directors of the National Dance Institute's Dance Barns and St. Elizabeth Shelter, a psychiatrist, two foster parents, a high school math teacher, and five more.

The psychiatrist, Lawrence Lazarus, Jane Clarke, a mental-health specialist who works with traumatized infants and their families, and Talitha Arnold, Senior Minister at the United Church of Santa Fe, have undergone years of academic training. The rest of the people you'll meet, though equally driven by their hearts, have gathered expertise pretty much on their own.

Every one of the book's thirteen chapters is an amalgam of five interviews, each lasting a couple of hours. The featured Good Samaritans answered half a dozen questions, ranging from "Tell us about what you do," to "What effect does religious or spiritual practice have on your work?" They were urged to enliven their answers with real-life for instances, thumbnail case histories and stories. In these we often decided to change real names and other details, though not the names of those interviewed.

Each chapter ends with a thumbnail bio, statistics related to the fields of activity, and useful websites, emails, regular mail addresses, and phones. All were accurate at the time of publication.

What we hope, dear reader, after finishing each chapter, is that you'll say to yourself three things:

> *Oh, I'm so glad I've gotten to know this person*, and
> *What a useful life*, and
> *Maybe I can find a few hours in a week to be helpful to others, too.*
>
> —Michael Scofield
> Santa Fe

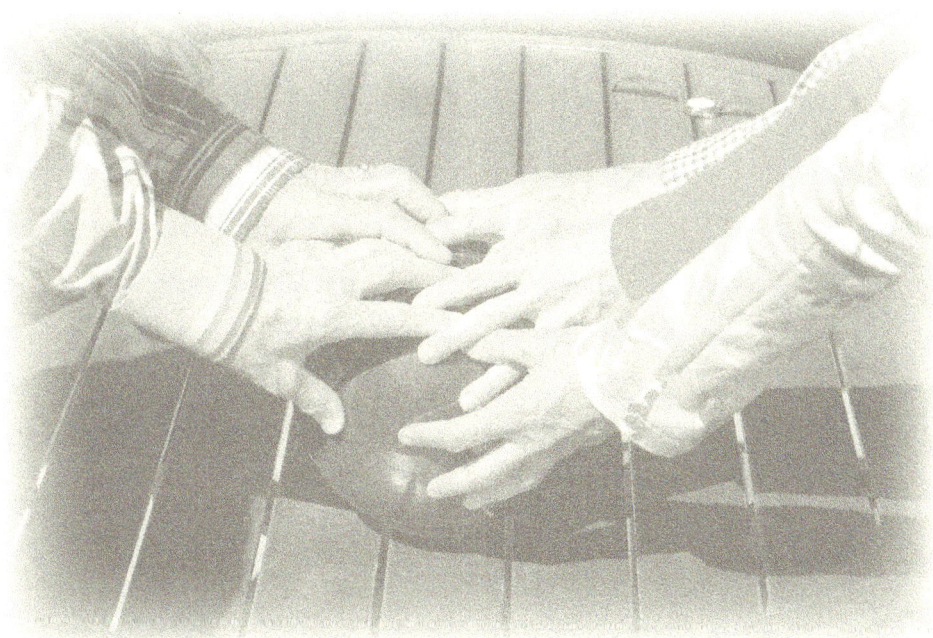

James McGrath
Teacher, Painter, Sculptor, Ceramist, Poet

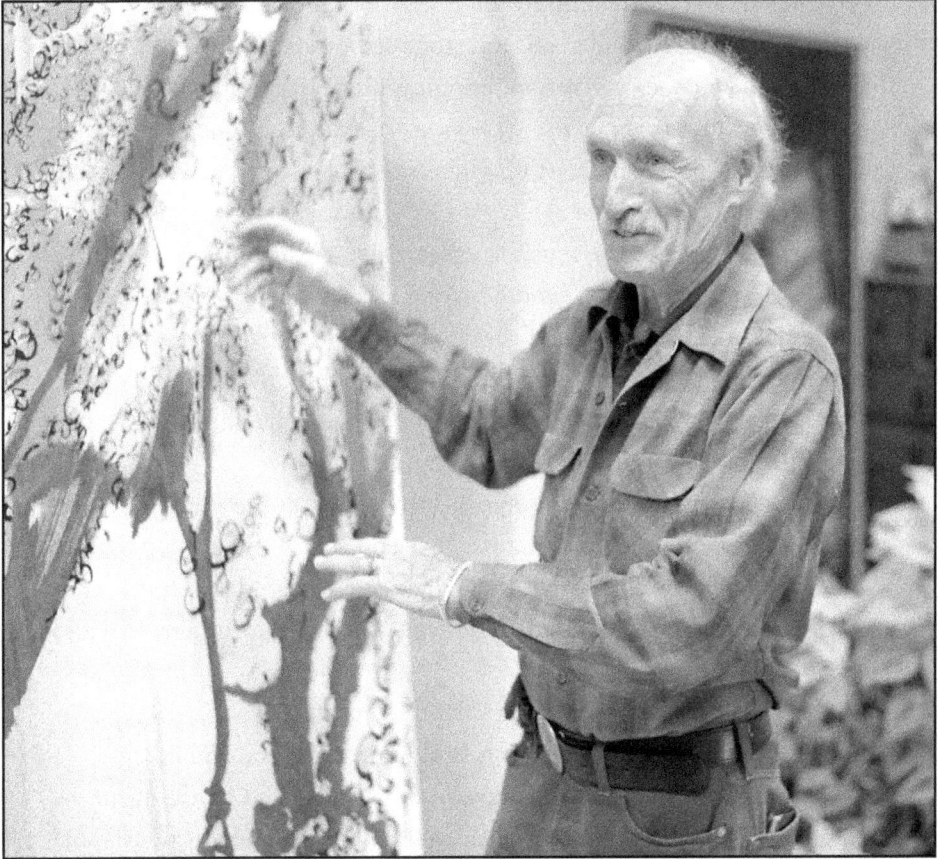

Q: James, tell us about your teaching activities.

A: Much of my work with young adults started in 1962, when I helped found the Institute of American Indian Arts (IAIA) in south Santa Fe, becoming an instructor, Assistant Art Director, Art Director, and then, for two years, Dean. Hopi teachers Charles and Otellie Loloma and I loved to spend weekends on the Hopi reservation north of Flagstaff to be inspired by the lifestyle and dances.

Before and after the IAIA experience, I went overseas to teach, but more about that later. Fast-forward to 1982. The principal at the Hopi Hotevilla-Bacavi School, kindergarten through eighth grade, asked me to develop an arts curriculum for ninety-seven kids, as well as teach clay, painting, drawing, stained glass, and stone sculpture. From 1982 to 1983 I spent a year on the reservation, bringing in local artisans to help. Our students won first prize at the statewide art exhibit. No one before had submitted paintings using earth pigments. At Christmas we staged Gian Carlo Menotti's *Amahl and the Night Visitors*, adding a Hopi wise man.

After my friend the music teacher, Robert Rhodes, had married a Hopi, he decided to start a school for the arts, held in various homes on the reservation, small classes of seven or eight kids, six adults. I've yearly taught for Robert the last two weeks in July, painting, drawing, clay. I've learned a few words in the men's language; women have their own. Thank you is kahkwah. Beautiful morning is loma talungva.

I've also taught a dozen seniors once a week at the Ponce de Leon Retirement Community in Santa Fe. They come with three ideas: that art should be representational, that they know what they like, and that they can't wait to learn the skills to show what they like to others. We also work on creative writing.

Here are ways I try to inspire them as artists:

I'll bring in fall leaves, squash, and pumpkins for a still life.

Maybe the next week I'll appear with baskets and fabrics from the Philippines. "It's cold in Santa Fe," I'll say. "Let's visit a warm country and paint what the locals are making."

Each spring when I've returned from the Writers Week in County Kerry, Ireland, I bring back postcards for them to interpret and poems to illustrate.

One week I'll display an Acoma pot and colored corn. Or give an assignment like, "Look out your room's window, sketch the view, then bring the sketch to class and paint it."

Once in a while we've gone outside to paint the plantings and goldfish.

At the end of the year, I put together a spiral-bound, full-color booklet of their art and writings. Everyone gets a copy.

From 1996 to 2002, year-around, New Mexico's Very Special Arts program asked five other artists and me to help physically and mentally challenged Albuquerque residents create artworks. I remember once we scoured nearby junkyards for fenders, bumpers, hood ornaments, car doors. The group drew spirals and arrows on the junk, and splashed it with bright colors. So much laughter, so childlike—while respecting each other's space. We bolted the parts into a couple of sculptures and installed them on the top level of the parking structure near the public library.

How I got involved with teaching outside of this country started at Columbia High School in Richland, Washington. After college I taught art there and oversaw production of the yearbook, 1952 to 1955. That last year, representatives from the Department of Defense (DOD) Dependent Schools Overseas came looking for K-12 instructors. I had a great yen to travel but not much money, so I signed up. In Europe I taught health and science as subjects for art at the Hanau American Elementary School. Drawings of intestines. Clay sculptures of kidneys. The students lived on military bases. Field trips to the Book Fair and Rapunzel's Tower, while teaching at Frankfurt American High School, were often the first time these kids had gone off base. Eventually I became Art Director for a hundred and eight DOD schools in Germany, France, and Italy.

After an eleven-year break to cofound and teach at IAIA, I agreed to another tour of duty with the DOD, this time for eleven years in the Far East, not including a year's break at Hopi. I lived in Japan, and traveled to South Korea, the Philippines, Taiwan, Okinawa, and Midway Island, finishing up as Art and Humanities Director for forty schools.

Five years later I hopped overseas again, this time for the State Department's Arts America program. We were sculptors, painters, poets, dancers, and musicians working with our indigenous counterparts for two to four weeks. In 1990 I traveled to Yemen, in 1992 to the Kingdom of Saudi Arabia, and in 1995 to the Republic of the Congo. I chose to use only local imagery and materials. Now the Smithsonian says it wants the eight thick scrapbooks I kept, documenting the projects.

Q: What life experiences have contributed to your doing this good work?

A: My parents only went through eighth grade but pretty much built our house in Tacoma, Washington, themselves. They raised me to stay very connected to nature, digging clams, for instance, and hunting deer.

From age two into college I lived summers with my aunt and Chehalis Indian uncle—no electricity or running water. In high school, Aunt Margaret taught me to paint watercolors of flowers and trees, and often took me to the Seattle Museum; it specialized in Asian art. Throughout high school I worked at my Uncle Art's high-end-design and furniture store afternoons.

The experience that inspires me to teach those with handicaps, mental or physical, is my own stuttering.

Stuttering since first grade had made me afraid to talk. The summer between eleventh and twelfth grade, however, I took speech correction, drama, painting, and drawing at Central Washington College of Education, now Central Washington University. Making art changed my life. I found I had gifts I hadn't known about, something people older than me saw the value of. I realized I could go to college, not stay in Tacoma and drive trucks for a living. I became more social, less withdrawn. I still stutter, but rarely.

Entering Central Washington as a freshman, I took every art class I could. My painting teacher, Sarah Spurgeon, was especially encouraging. She had a low, warm voice. I can still see her in a loose smock, tall, white hair all piled up. She always displayed our works for others to admire.

After two years, I transferred to the University of Oregon because it offered a broader selection of courses in the arts.

My later, around-the-world travels taught me that all of us—young, old, disabled or well, wealthy, poor—have the need to show how we live, what food we cook, stories we like, how we care for each other or don't.

I treat my groups like communities, encourage everyone to express themselves as individuals but also to acknowledge that the artworks of others are equally important. I believe that all people are born creative but that life squelches our potential. Mostly as a teacher I wish to help you realize what you're capable of.

When I taught art at Columbia High School, and later overseas and at IAIA, I never knew if students' best efforts were going to be visual, so I'd bring in poetry, music, dance, even examples of architecture to be inspired by.

I know it worked because, at the time of the publication of this book, I'm still in touch, by letter and telephone, with some students. Jim Scoggin is an architect in San Rafael, California, William Witherup is a published poet in Seattle, John Haugse is a filmmaker in Hood River, Oregon. Christine Patten in Vadito, New Mexico, sells her drawings for upwards of ten thousand dollars, Donna Salazar is a ceramist in Española, David Montana is a modern dancer on the Papago reservation in Arizona, William Wylie was honored in 2010 by a retrospective of his paintings at the Smithsonian American Art Museum. They keep sending me gifts of their work.

The inspiration for teaching art skills to elders is my mother. She died at ninety-six in the house where I grew up. When she developed dementia at age ninety, I came to visit before Christmas. "Mom," I asked, "would you like to make some greeting cards?" Though she used to crochet and bake cookies, she'd never learned visual-arts techniques.

"Sure!" she said. "Why not?"

We had a ball making potato prints of ornaments, trees, and toys.

Q: Any role models who inspire you?

A: I think of three. My partner, Daniel Forest, is a massage therapist in Albuquerque. On weekends he comes to Santa Fe or I drive down.

Both of us do ink-brush calligraphy, write poetry, garden, hike. We cook together and sometimes dance around the kitchen. He's a good listener and this motivates me creatively—we cross-fertilize each other.

Cynthia West, a longtime friend, and I attend pueblo dances dawn to dusk and express these experiences on paper and canvas. We also write together, as well as derive inspiration from spending time in each other's gardens. Her openness and creative honesty energizes my own.

Some years ago Billie Morris started art classes with me at Ponce de Leon. She'd had no training but has become one of my most accomplished students by painting between classes. She's found a new way of getting to know herself, she says, which supports my teaching philosophy, that every one of us has a unique artistic need.

Q: How do you arrange the rest of your life to do this good work?

A: I try to budget enough time for several other kinds of activities.

First, time for lunches out, museum visits, readings in my apple orchard for local writers, telephone calls to old friends in Ireland and Greece, letter writing by hand—I don't own a computer and can no longer find ribbons for my college typewriter.

Secondly, I take care in preparing for my classes, gathering materials, coming up with ideas for students' paintings or drawings or sculptures, doing everything I can to ensure their comfort in the space we'll be using, in order to promote their trust in me as an instructor.

Thirdly, I always set aside time for post-class evaluation. Not just how did I do today as a teacher, but also, how did Billie respond? Did Rob and Beverly enjoy the class? Do I think students acquired respect for their own and the others' works? Will the rest of the school or retirement community get to see the art pieces in hallways or on walls?

Q: What effect does religious or spiritual practice have on your work?

A: Every day I'm surrounded by the natural world: rocks, fruit trees, cottonwoods, magpies, hawks, foxes, raccoons, the neighbors' horses and cows, the Santa Fe River forming one boundary of my eight acres. I live in a three-hundred-year-old, former stagecoach stop, now powered by solar energy. There are six fireplaces for heat and a windmill for water.

Plus I meditate, but not like most people. Every other week I practice the tea ceremony, edo senkei, which takes an hour. After seven years' study in Japan and Okinawa, I received my certificate to teach tea. For four years I also studied flower arranging, sogetso. I create two arrangements a week. And once in a while I practice shodo, ink-brush calligraphy.

My environment and meditation practices give me a sense of peace, strengthen my conviction that there are important realities besides human beings. In my travels I learned about Shinto, Islam, Buddhism, the Native American way of life, Taoism, shamanism, and others. In all these there seems to be a base of kindness and community, which I try to bring into my teaching.

Q: What doubts and disappointments have you had to deal with?

A: My biggest past doubt is having taken so much time away from family life that after nine years of marriage from right out of college, my wife, Jean, divorced me while I was serving as Art Director in Karlsruhe, Germany. She had taken our daughters, Jain and Jeni, back to Portland, Oregon, and I came to Santa Fe to help get IAIA off the ground.

Part of me is sad that I've no current interest in producing visual art, or adding art-teaching jobs to what I've got. I turned down an offer to introduce earth-pigment painting for a fall workshop hosted by the art museum in Roswell. But I want to be free in my later years to do what I feel like, when to go to town, when to sleep, when to climb a tree—why not?

Yet I always need a way in the arts to express myself. So I'm writing poems about the natural world's beauty, wars and global warming, Jeni's August death from cancer at age sixty-two, my own death.

As far as disappointments go, the biggest is that over the decades I put so much energy into teaching that I had relatively little left for my own creativity.

Two disappointments took place in the Far East, the first on an American military base in Seoul, South Korea. I'd hired locals to teach grades one through six. The school's principal had asked me to come up with a mural for a fifty-foot hallway wall. I picked animals from the Korean zodiac like the dragon, the monkey, and the tiger. Students made stencils and used acrylics to apply the colors.

But one of the base's Christian ministers called us blasphemous for painting Buddhist images. America was a Christian culture, he said, and ours was a Christian school. Remove the mural, he told me. When I refused, the school hired painters to cover our wall in gallbladder green.

Another incident ended in my taking leave for a year. As the DOD schools' Far East Art Director, I'd started an artist-in-residence program for forty schools, bringing over dancers, jewelers, poets, printmakers, sculptors, architects, storytellers, even a juggler from the United States, to visit six to eight schools for two weeks each.

I once gave an architect from Oregon the mission to improve her assigned schools' environments by getting teachers and students to work on landscaping and murals, and on rearranging room interiors for more effective learning. She shared that she'd set up a system with the university to give university credit to all the American teachers she'd be working with. Exciting, I thought.

But when I told the Assistant Curriculum Director, she responded, "Oh, those fly-by-night colleges. Why do we want one of them involved?"

I lost my temper, and received a reprimand from the DOD schools' director. He arranged for me to take a year off. That's when I went to live and teach on the Hopi reservation.

Meanwhile, the architect, a caring human being, did a first-rate job, and got the teachers their credits at the university.

Q: Will you share a couple of your successes?

A: In 1962, a seventeen-year-old Crow Indian from Lodge Grass, Montana, Kevin Red Star, was one of the first to enroll at IAIA. We were in the midst of construction—holding art classes in the bakery and storing paintings in the ovens. In Kevin's desire to create from his Crow culture I sensed a lot of talent. We worked together for three years.

Early on Kevin brought me samples of Crow beadwork on shirts and moccasins. I told him, "Use these patterns but enlarge them in a different way, after looking into your heart and your culture and your personal DNA."

The results were breakthroughs for him and for Indian works in general. He produced canvases as large as four feet by six, shields, breastplates, dancers, individuals, sometimes layering on colors so thick the paintings seemed bas-reliefs. After graduation he received a full scholarship to the San Francisco Art Institute.

In 2014 Gibbs Smith Publishers came out with a hundred and ninety-one page, four-color book of Kevin's work. Well, I thought, seeing the book, I did something right.

Off and on, from 1987 through 1997, I taught visual arts and writing in many of our schools, K through twelve, for New Mexico's Arts Division. An outstanding success occurred at Tularosa Elementary, near Three Rivers Petroglyph State Park. After seeing the petroglyphs, fourth and sixth graders hammered images of airplanes, horses, dogs, and cats into large rocks scattered around the school yard. They shaped wax sculptures of their representations and had them cast in bronze. By means of welded rods, they embedded these sculptures in the same large rocks.

Meanwhile, second, third, and fourth graders created, fired, and glazed life-size clay sculptures of rabbits and prairie dogs for the yard.

Their teachers surrounded these and the rocks with cactus, chamisa, Apache plume, and penstemon. The school yard became their park. The project took six weeks. To celebrate, some kids dressed up as crows, others wore sunflower headdresses; we marched around while the 'crows' cawed. To finish off, I invited all sixty kids and their parents to a full day's workshop. They painted a mural with earth pigments and created miniature clay sculptures of local animals: horses, cows, sheep, llamas, ostriches, and, of course, dogs and cats.

Q: What tips can you pass on for successful fund-raising?

A: I've been fortunate to receive grants from several sources: the DOD schools, the National Endowment for the Arts, and New Mexico's Arts Division, including its Very Special Arts, activities for the mentally and physically challenged.

I've found it's important, in making grant proposals, to be clear, be concise, and use small, easily understood words in describing the project and the community it hopes to serve.

Here are other things to consider:

Listing past-project successes usually is a good idea. So is sharing your passion for the current project.

Be sure to outline exactly what monies you need and why, as well as detailing the outcomes expected. Always include an up-to-date resumé and references.

It helps to get funds if you promise to produce an evaluation report after your project has ended. In that report, the grant-making agency usually is grateful for suggestions on how it might further the impact of your project by offering additional grants.

James McGrath's Thumbnail Bio:

Born in Tacoma, Washington, 1928. BS, University of Oregon, 1950; MA, University of New Mexico, 1973. High school art teacher, 1952–1955. Department of Defense (DOD) Overseas School Division, teacher, then Art Director, Europe, 1955–1962; Far East, 1973–1982. Art teacher, US State Department's Arts America program: Yemen, 1990; Saudi Arabia, 1992; Congo, 1995. Cofounder, Institute of American Indian Arts (IAIA); instructor, Assistant Art Director, then Art Director, 1962–1973; Dean, 1988–1990. Art teacher on Hopi reservation full-time, 1983; two weeks every July, since 2000. Art and creative writing teacher at Ponce de Leon Retirement Community, Santa Fe, New Mexico, since 2000. Art exhibits: Bellevue, Washington, 1952; thirty exhibits worldwide, 1953–2014; fifty-year retrospective, Meridian Gallery, San Francisco, California, 2015. Five books of poetry, Sunstone Press, 2004–2014. Designated a Santa Fe Living Treasure, 2008.

To Get Help

If you'd like to learn or hone an artistic skill, here are contacts:

National

> American Society of Artists
> PO Box 1326
> Palatine, IL 60078
> (312) 751-2500
> www.americansocietyofartists.us

> The Art Institutes
> 210 Sixth Avenue, 33rd Floor
> Pittsburgh, PA 15222
> (888) 624-0300
> www.visit.artinstitutes.edu

> American Art Therapy Association
> 4875 Eisenhower Avenue, Suite 240
> Alexandria, VA 22304

(continued)

(888) 290-0878
www.arttherapy.org

In Santa Fe

Santa Fe Convention and Visitors Bureau
210 W. Marcy Ave.
Santa Fe, NM 87501
(505) 955-6200
www.santafe.org/classes and workshops

Santa Fe Children's Museum
1050 Old Pecos Trail
Santa Fe, NM 87505
(505) 989-8359
www.santafechildrensmuseum.org

Annabelle Montoya
Former Northeastern Regional Manager, New Mexico Chapter, Alzheimer's Association

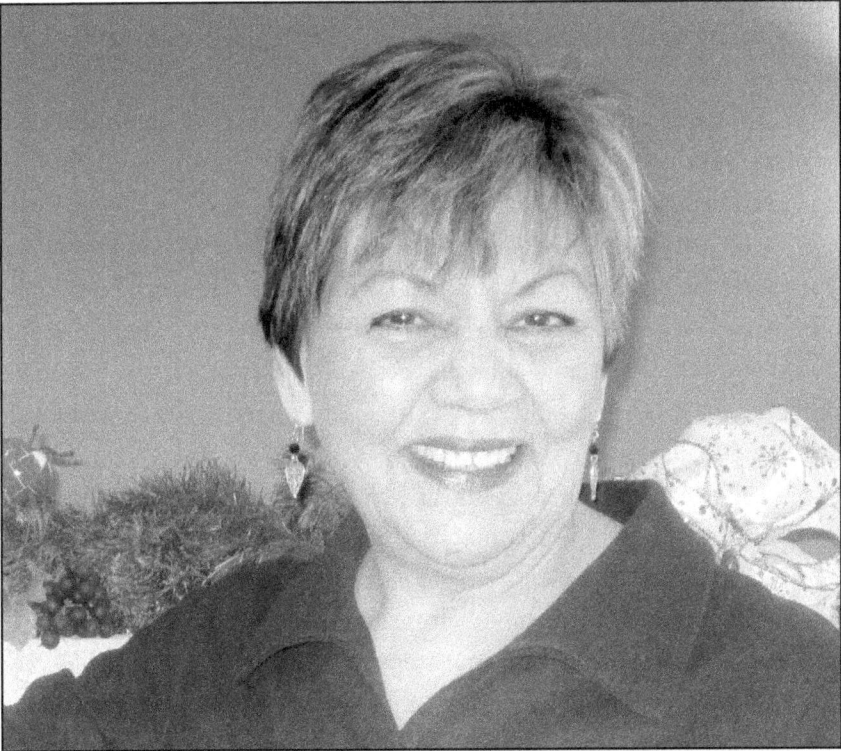

Q: Annabelle, tell us about your duties.

A: Mostly I reassure caregivers in Taos, Los Alamos, Santa Fe, and points east that they don't have to go through their dire times alone. Dementia is not a mental illness, it's a disease of the brain that ends in death. The Association can help financially, however, and we have classes, support groups, and a resource library.

Using what I've learned from twenty-four hours of intensive training in Albuquerque, and update courses monthly, I consult with maybe a thousand caregivers a year. These caregivers represent over four hundred sufferers.

In one class I showed a husband how to rephrase. He and his wife planned to watch Zozobra burn from the balcony of friends. Though they'd never visited these friends, his wife kept insisting they had. Instead of correcting her, he learned simply to say, "We're going to have so much fun."

The caregiver needs to understand: don't force, don't argue, don't try to make your loved one remember. She or he will mirror your behavior. You need to stay calm.

Like caregivers, the persons afflicted are doing the best they can. They're not being angry or stubborn or lazy. The disease—dead brain cells, tangles and plaques—is in control, and it can start twenty years before the first symptoms. The personality changes. The ability to plan, to organize thoughts, to execute familiar tasks, to access memories accurately—all become threatening.

Think of what's happening like this: normal aging is going from one room to another, forgetting why, retracing your steps, then remembering. A famous actor said, "As I get older, I get more exercise than ever." Dementia is different. It's going from one room to another, forgetting why, and forgetting to retrace your steps.

Often I hear from a family member or other caregiver, "Annabelle, we were doing everything wrong." For instance, I'd not yet had a chance to counsel two sisters whose older sister had Alzheimer's. Because the older sister volunteered at the church, a younger sister asked her to speak about an upcoming fund-raiser. When she got in front of the podium, she said something like this:

"Good morning, everybody, how's everything? I'm up here to tell you that we're having a wonderful event. I don't know what it is, I don't know when, or where, or why."

Afterward the younger sister lashed out, "What's the matter with you? Are you crazy? What the heck were you saying up there?"

Q: What life experiences have contributed to your doing this good work?

A: Being raised by a loving mother and father, and experiencing how they died. They came down from Tierra Amarilla in Northern New Mexico. We were fourteen kids, become ten, living in a three-bedroom home. If I had to use our one bathroom, a sister or brother would say, "Sure, I'll let you go first but you have to do the dishes for a week."

My parents were always the ones to help people in need. I don't remember them ever gossiping or being judgmental. When I was thirty or thirty-two, I said, "Mama, how do you do this all the time, helping out, and so many who don't appreciate it?"

"Mi hija," she said, "I do it because I want to, not because I expect anything in return."

That stopped me in my tracks. It was a redirection. I realized there's a different dance for everyone.

Mama died in 1994 of bone cancer. First she was misdiagnosed with osteoarthritis, maybe because she started carrying her left arm in her right. You could see the pain on her face. But her death, like my dad's, served as a spiritual experience. She talks to me all the time.

After the correct diagnosis came, all ten of us gathered in the house. Mama gave each of us individual guidance for when she'd be gone. I thought I'd never forget her words, but I have. Two months later, my sister, Vita, called. "Choo-Choo," she said, "better come." Maybe because I didn't want to be there, I arrived late from taking a shower. But I was in time to say goodbye. Mama opened her eyes to make sure we were all there, and took her last breath.

A man of few words, my father died a few years later of congestive heart failure, at age eighty-eight. In his bed at Christus St. Vincent

Hospital he told me, "Choo-Choo, I've lived a beautiful life. I love you all very much, and I want you to stay united"—though sadly we haven't. "I'm not leaving you much but at least I'm not leaving you in debt."

Daddy had dug potatoes, been a shipbuilder in San Francisco, a bus driver in Chama, and then worked for New Mexico's Department of Motor Vehicles. I know I was his favorite—but all his kids say the same thing.

How my parents died, grateful for life and for us, led me to want to be a caregiver. So did the death of my longtime employer, Philip Naumburg. He died of non-Hodgkin's lymphoma a year after Mama. I started with his company, Colony Materials Ready-Mix, as receptionist and ended up twenty-five years later as CEO. We had over one-hundred employees and sales of twelve million a year.

Philip allowed me the luxury, in fact, demanded, that I get involved in community services. After he passed, I sold the company for his wife, and used my parachute to found La Vida Hermosa, a fourteen-bed as-sisted-living home. My sister, Rose, and I financed it fifty/fifty, though it turned out we had different ideas on how to treat people. In 2007 I sold my half to her.

I think I've always had a passion to help others. Growing up on West San Francisco Street, we had a couple of folks who liked to drink too much. They used to sit in the dirt against a wall. I'd make them pot-ted-meat or egg-salad sandwiches—I was only seven or eight. Though Mama was afraid I'd get hurt, she said, "You will never lack for anything because you're always giving." It's when I'm happiest. Five years ago, one of the neighbor kids, grown up, asked me, "Do you remember when you'd put on puppet shows for my eleven siblings and me, and we'd laugh and sing?"

Q: Any current role models who inspire you?

A: My older sister, Dora. She was the first Hispanic Senior Vice President in banking in Santa Fe without a college degree. Her bank let her become involved in community services—United Way, cooking pancakes on the Fourth of July at the Plaza. She produced managers because she brought out the best in people. And she was so encouraging to me.

Ben Baca, too. Even with his chemo and oxygen tank, he helped eight young adults get their GEDs in 2013. "You deserve to walk in your cap and gown," he told them. I loved being around this guy. He's worked with special-ed children and in prison ministries.

Q: How do you arrange the rest of your life to let you do this work?

A: If you talked to my family, they might say, "She's so busy doing things for others, she doesn't have time for us." If my husband or one of my children or siblings is in need, I'm right there. If no one's in need, then yes, I'm off doing my thing. As well as earning a living by it, I'm the Alzheimer Association's best volunteer. And I volunteer my family.

My mind never stops. If I say, "I've got an idea," everybody's afraid. In conversations, people have a hard time keeping up. I come on too strong, maybe. In former days I was pretty intimidating.

It used to be the more I did, the more I could do. People asked, "How do you find the time?" I'm still busy but everything takes me longer. I used to drive others crazy because I wanted it all done yesterday. Now I'm more of a procrastinator, though I still excel under pressure—best at the midnight hour.

When I was younger, it was easier to keep the plates spinning. My greatest hobby was, and is, to cook and to bake—enchiladas, chocolate cakes. One of my kids' favorites is Chicken a la Suisse. I still love to give parties: Halloween, Chinese, Moulin Rouge, Mardi Gras, Dolce Vita, Christmas, Valentine's Day, Hawaii. I also give friends and family blankets, two sheets of fleece tied together with colored strips of fleece, for watching TV or reading. Collecting Hispanic tinwork, straw art, bultos, and retablos remains a major pleasure. Many of the artists are my friends.

I used to walk every day. During the stress of selling La Vida Hermosa, I gained weight. But guess who walks beside the Alzheimer's truck in the Historical/Hysterical parade? All my friends are decrepit: bad hips, knees, backs, hearts. They ride. I, who shouldn't walk, do walk, handing out fliers—and my left Achillies tendon flares up.

Less and less have I time for doing things I don't like to do. I think I'm wiser in this and accepting myself more. For instance, I used to be brutally honest. If you asked me out for lunch, I might have said, "That's the last restaurant I'd like to go to." Now I say, "No thank you," or suggest an alternative.

Q: What effect does religious or spiritual practice have on your work?

A: I'm just an instrument of the Holy Spirit. When I go into a classroom to teach, I ask Him to come in, too, knowing He'll offer comfort and guidance, empathy and generosity. He'll eliminate judgment and criticism.

I go to Mass every Sunday. My husband and I attend weekend Cursillos to renew our faith—no radios, no phones. And we help out with the church's Marriage Enrichment Program, believing it's a triangle: husband, wife, God.

Here are a few of my simple prayers. "Help me." "Thank You." "I love You." Plus, "I know I'm Your favorite, even though I know You love everyone."

Q: Will you share a couple of your disappointments in carrying out your good work?

A: It's financially, physically, and emotionally devastating for someone as caregiver to go on the Alzheimer's journey, knowing you are going to lose your loved one. Yet most of us were brought up to take care of our own. There's a lot of stigma and shame in calling for help. The Association can simplify caregivers' lives but they have to make themselves known. So many of them don't.

Another disappointment is that the Association's financial goals keep increasing, meaning I have to spend more and more time raising funds, and less and less on our true mission, to be helpful. The criteria for getting grant money from the state and from Chicago headquarters—I mean the number of caregivers I need to assist—is often too high, impractical.

Q: What doubts do you deal with in your work?

A: That I might overstep my boundaries, make wrong assumptions. I have to remember I'm an outsider. I only know from a professional's standpoint what caregivers are going through. I don't have their grief or sense of loss or pain. Sometimes I'm afraid I make solutions sound easy.

Once in a while I deal with my own shame. Two years ago I was helping a woman find ways to care for her father. Already she had set up assisted-living in his home. For the round-the-clock caregivers and medical assistants, she'd placed chewing gum, playing cards, and harmonicas in an old violin case of his. She, herself, sang for him and told jokes.

But he developed an obsession, every few minutes calling out, "I have to go wee-wee." Doctors couldn't understand why. The woman was in a panic. I told her I'd present the case in the monthly class I take, taught by doctors at the University of New Mexico. She started calling me twenty times a day. Finally she bypassed me and contacted the physician who led the class. I lost my cool—my brother-in-law was dying. I shouted at her on the phone. We later apologized but my behavior still bothers me. Her father's problem turned out to be kidney cancer.

I have another doubt. Am I getting too old to be working with young people? Because my generation can live without an iPhone, they think we're dumb, they expect us to agree with everything they say. Just a month ago I called a staff member in Albuquerque to place a full-color ad for the annual Alzheimer's Walk fund-raiser. She indicated there was no hurry by saying, "Not happening." So I went to our events coordinator and the ad got placed in time. "No" is not in my vocabulary.

How do I relieve my doubts? I pray. At the end of the day I tell myself I'm only human and so is everyone else. And I choose my battles.

Q: How about examples of your successes?

A: One of the brothers of a family of six who were caregivers for their mom called me. I met him at a truck stop in Española and, because all worked, I arranged for an evening meeting. During the three-hour presentation in the midst of a thunderstorm—oh, the booms—I explained that good caregivers care for themselves first. I said that they needn't feel guilty, that, while trying to be loving, of course they're afraid of the disease, afraid it will destroy family bonds. And I laid out sources of financial aid and other kinds of support.

Soon they started feeling more comfortable sharing vulnerabilities and their too-high expectations of themselves and of the Alzheimer's sufferer. Later they realized that having a damaged loved one to care for was not the end of the road, just a different journey. When I left, they said they felt to be on the same page, far more compassionate of Mom and toward each other.

Recently a woman and her husband—him a bit over eighty and just diagnosed with Alzheimer's—came in for a consultation. He was healthy in other ways, very kind, concerned for his wife, but confused. I told her that the more she could make eye contact with him, the more he would feel at ease, that because he can't come into our reality, she needed to try to come into his.

They each have three children, and hoped to make realistic plans for the future. It was important to her to include his wishes, but the more we talked about financial concerns, medical emergencies, and end-of-life, the more she realized it was she who would be making plans. Later she attended my Savvy Caregiver class and became an ongoing member of my support group. The next step, a good one, is a consultation involving the six children.

Q: How do you go about fund-raising?

A: You have to believe you're going to meet your goal. And with everyone I meet, I try to talk about how the Alzheimer's Association can help those in need.

Much of the credit for reaching our goal goes to my events committee, nine women and three men. One works for a reverse-mortgage company, the others for home-care services and assisted-living facilities. Such enthusiasm! We're caregivers to each other. This year we'll stage six to nine fund-raisers. Before each we hold two to four weekly meetings, a couple of hours in the afternoon. I donate the snacks: hummus, salsa, crackers, brownies, and cheese.

One afternoon all we did was laugh, brainstorming themes for our float. Outrageous. But we needed that. This kind of work takes its toll.

My territory's two big events are the Caregiver Conference in July and the Walk to End Alzheimer's in Railyard Park in September. I talk them up in my Savvy Caregiver classes, at senior centers, in doctors' offices and hospitals. And I post flyers. This year my youngest son, Matt, sent emails and made phone calls to those who'd attended previous classes.

The Caregivers Conference is free, eight a.m. to four p.m. We provide a continental breakfast and catered lunch, this year vegetarian pasta or chicken stuffed with cranberries and Brie. At registration we gave out a tote bag marked *Alzheimer's* filled with a pen, water bottle, mug, a clip for potato-chip bags, and a key chain, each imprinted with a different sponsor's name.

For the first time we set aside a Breathing Room, to pamper caregivers: massage, Reike hands-over-body work to revive energy, applications of Mary Kay cosmetics for the women, even nail polishing. The keynote speaker was Lena Smith, a PhD and the CEO of Retreat Healthcare. Breakout-session titles included "Money Matters," "Caregiving: the Good, the Bad, and the Ugly," "Legal Matters," and "Taking Care of Yourself." Home-care and assisted-living representatives sat at tables to answer questions during breaks. We all left rejuvenated.

The September Walk to End Alzheimer's drew probably three hundred people in 2014. Everyone was encouraged to wear purple. My husband, Adolfo, filled in as master of ceremonies. Son Joe sold raffle tickets at one dollar each. My oldest, Steve, and other volunteers served a breakfast of burritos or scrambled eggs. We marched the half mile around Railyard Park while Matt snapped photographs. Afterwards, Adolfo read out winning raffle tickets. Pre-Walk fund-raisers and the Walk itself raised $35,400, exceeding the Association's goal.

Other ways we've raised money? A motorcycle rally in October, a pancake breakfast at Ponce de Leon Senior Living, a bunch of rummage sales, an enchilada dinner, and auctioning off one of Liberace's white pianos at Kingston Residence. At one in my office's parking lot I noticed a man, maybe in his thirties, hunched on a bench with a bedroll and bag beside him. "Come help yourself," I said, pointing to the pizzas, salads, lemonade, and tea that Adolfo had brought us. He walked over, joined us for lunch, took out his wallet, and handed me a dollar. "It's not much. But this is a good cause." I couldn't reject it. I had to honor his dignity.

Annabelle Montoya's Thumbnail Bio:

Born in Santa Fe, 1949. CEO of Colony Materials, Inc. (ready-mix concrete), 1970–1996. Graduated from Santa Fe Business College, 1972. Cofounder of La Vida Hermosa 14-bed assisted-living home, 1998–2007. Assistant General Manager, Rainbow Vision, 2008–2009. Northeastern Regional Manager for Alzheimer's Association New Mexico, 2011–present. President: Literary Volunteers of Santa Fe. Cofounder: People of Color AIDS Foundation. President: Naumburg Adult Learning Center. Business Woman of the Year, 1992. One of Ten Who Made a Difference in Santa Fe, 1996.

Statistics on Alzheimer's Disease:

The most common type of dementia, Alzheimer's, is a progressive brain disorder. There is no known cause or cure. Symptoms include memory loss, impaired judgment, increasing problems with routine tasks, disorientation, and loss of language skills. Six in ten victims will wander. In New Mexico, 31,000 have contracted the disease. They have 105,000 family members and friends who provide unpaid care.

Nationally, an estimated 5.2 million people have Alzheimer's. Approximately five million of these are over 65. That works out to one in nine Americans who host the disease, but half, according to the Alzheimer's Association's *2014 Facts and Figures*, may not know it.

To Help Out, Or Get Help

To join a support group, participate in fund-raising walks, take classes for caregivers, use regional Alzheimer's Association libraries, request financial aid, or participate in conferences, make contact as follows:

National Office for Alzheimer's Association

> 225 N. Michigan Avenue, Floor 17
> Chicago, IL 60601-7633
> 24/7 helpline: (800) 272-3900
> www.alz.org

New Mexico Offices for Alzheimer's Association

9500 Montgomery Blvd. NE, Suite 121
Albuquerque, NM 87111
(505) 266-4473

Farmington (505) 326-3680
Las Cruces (575) 647-3868
Roswell (575) 624-1552
Santa Fe (505) 473-1297

www.alz.org/newmexico

Lawrence Lazarus, MD
Geriatric Psychiatrist

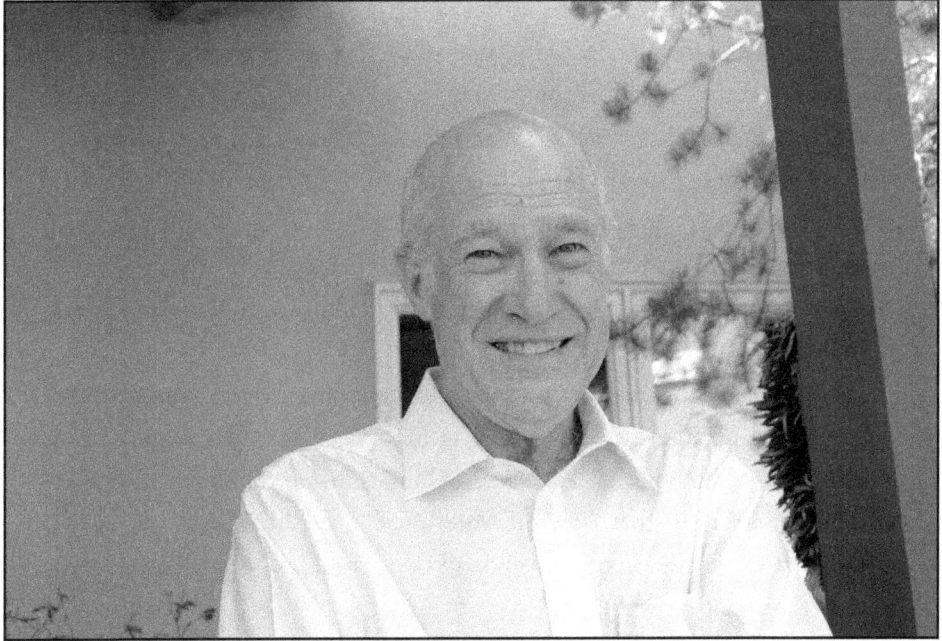

Q: Larry, tell us what you do.

A: Since I'm in the latter stages of my career, I see maybe ten to twelve patients a week, Monday mornings and all day Tuesday, leaving time for other interests—I'll expand on this later. I have forty to fifty patients all told, fourteen- to nearly ninety-years old. Most of them I see weekly, some every few months. Probably two-thirds are women. I'll make a house call if an elderly patient can't come to the office.

From 1980 to 2000, when I left Chicago for Santa Fe, I was seeing as many as fifty patients a week, a hundred-plus patients in all, at my office, in the hospital, and in nursing homes. The types of illnesses I treat are still pretty much the same as then: depression, psychiatric complications from dementia, phobic disorders like social anxiety and claustrophobia, and substance abuse.

To maximize healing, it's crucial for physicians in general and psychiatrists in particular to understand the whole patient. A while back I worked with a woman in her sixties who'd grown dependent on hydrocodone, prescribed by her physician for chronic pain after she broke her arm. I prescribed suboxone to help her taper off—it's less addictive. I saw her for half an hour every three weeks for a year and a half. Along the way she did some foolish things. She stopped the suboxone without telling me and ended up suffering withdrawal symptoms: sweating, nausea, pain in her legs, anxiety, excessive fatigue. Another time she increased the dose, not telling me, and ran out of the medication before our next appointment.

At the end of treatment, free from suboxone, she asked to give me a hug, and I decided to let her. She wanted to express her appreciation that I hadn't fired her, that I'd stayed willing to listen to details about her troubled marriage—that I seemed interested in her life. I *was* interested; I like to stick with patients through all their troubles because so often it speeds their getting well.

What pleases me most is finding a simple way to ease a patient's suffering. A retired accountant, who relocated from Chicago, began stressing out adapting to Santa Fe's laid-back lifestyle. He'd gotten used to long-term relationships with old-fashioned doctors, but here discovered he'd have to wait three months to see a primary care physician—or be turned down altogether. His stomach upsets and chest pains worsened. In our second session he worried that, like several of his friends, he was due for a heart attack.

I called a colleague specializing in internal medicine, who agreed to see my patient within a few days. The stomach upsets and chest pains disappeared. My phone call turned out to be faster-acting and less expensive than prescribing a tranquilizer like lorazepam or clonazepam.

One of my specialties is forensic psychiatry, that is, helping to appraise someone's mental state for the courts. A common challenge is determining an older person's capacity to execute or change a will. Six months ago a lawyer asked me to assess a former chain-store CEO's mental competence to alter his will, leaving more money than before to a blood son and daughter.

He had recently married a woman thirty-seven years younger, and made out a will leaving most of his estate to her. His son and daughter, about his wife's age, cried foul. You might be interested in some of the questions I asked as he approached his ninety-second birthday.

1. Do you know the names and relationships of family members?

2. Please describe the nature and extent of your estate. Also describe the professional who manages it.

3. What is your rationale for wanting to write a new will?

I double-checked with his children the accuracy of his responses, as well as critiqued his overall physical and mental status.

Meanwhile, the wife—with two kids of her own—hired her own lawyer. He, in turn, hired a psychiatrist who, after examining the man, submitted a report like mine. The two lawyers negotiated and concluded, based on our reports, that the man was indeed fit to change his will.

So this case, like most, did not have to go to trial—time-consuming, emotionally draining, and very expensive. And the marriage survived.

Q: What life experiences contributed to your becoming a psychiatrist?

A: Early on, my parents started taking my sister and me to plays, concerts, and ballets at Brooklyn College, a miniature Santa Fe in terms of how many cultural events it offered the public. The arts, in my opinion, are expressions of character development and human relationships. Ellen and I also followed our parents' lead as voracious readers. As a teenager I became fascinated by how novelists revealed the psychological states of their protagonists. At college I majored in American and English literature, intensifying my fascination with human behavior.

Between 1963 and 1967, at Drexel Medical College in Philadelphia, the training director in psychiatry was Dr. Paul Fink. Later he chaired the psych department at Temple University, and after that was elected president of the American Psychiatric Association, which now has more than thirty-six-thousand members. While I was treating an especially difficult schizophrenic patient, Dr. Fink said he thought I had the aptitude to become a fine psychiatrist. On graduation another student and I won the Psychiatry Prize.

My three-year residency took place at Chicago's Michael Reese Medical Center. In those days, the focus of training was how best to apply psychoanalytic theory. This was way before biological psychiatry—the prescribing of meds for major and minor disorders—became prominent. Our supervisors were psychoanalysts; meds were a small part of our training.

During our residency a fellow student asked me to assist in developing group therapy and other programs for those over sixty-five. In 1978, seven years following graduation, a few others and I helped him start the American Association for Geriatric Psychiatry, currently fourteen hundred members strong.

Q: Any current role models who inspire you?

A: Dr. Jan Fawcett, at age eighty-two, is professor of psychiatry at the University of New Mexico. He recently headed an international team of psychiatrists to update the mood-disorders section of the *Diagnostic and Statistical Manual* (*DSM-5*) of the American Psychiatric Association. This is the world's bible for the classification of psychiatric disorders.

For twenty-three years, starting about 1977, Jan chaired the psychiatry department at Rush Medical College in Chicago, where I directed the Geriatric Psychiatry Fellowship Program. He's a renowned teacher and researcher in depression, suicide, and psychopharmacology.

We weren't especially close yet. Fourteen years ago, without knowing the other planned to do so, Jan and I moved to Santa Fe. At the time of this book's publication we meet monthly for dinner at Harry's Roadhouse, where I discuss, without naming them, a few of my more challenging patients because, even though I'm seventy-three, I continue to find it valuable to hone my skills with a more experienced mentor.

Jan is a generous man with a huge range of interests. For several years he volunteered at Santa Fe's La Familia Medical Center. Some years ago he learned how to pilot a glider off nearby mountaintops. He has read at Collected Works Bookstore and Coffeehouse in Santa Fe from his novel, *Living Forever*. He's wiry, probably five foot eight, and has a wide smile, an excellent sense of humor, and a full head of white hair.

Q: You mentioned wanting to make time for other interests. Please explain.

A: I like to contribute to the aggregate health of whatever community I live in. For instance, in 2011, I put together a directory to help primary care physicians and other health professionals refer patients to the most appropriate psychiatrists in Santa Fe. What insurance, if any, do they take; who combines psychotherapy with pharmacotherapy; who practices forensic psychiatry; who specializes in alcohol and drug abuse; who concentrates on couples, families, children, adults, or seniors? The information's all in there. I hope to add an edition of it to existing websites, such as that of the New Mexico Medical Society (www.nmms.org) and the Psychiatric Medical Association of New Mexico (www.pmanm.org).

Supporting the arts is another key interest. For several years I served as a docent at the New Mexico Museum of Art. I like to lend paintings for special exhibitions to museums throughout the state. I've pledged a few thousand dollars to the School of the Aspen Santa Fe Ballet to help fund scholarships for young dancers.

Tennis and three days a week at the gym are important. I also like to travel. In addition, I hope to do more interviews about, and more public readings from my book, *Getting the Health Care You Deserve in America's Broken Health Care System*, self-published in 2013.

In the free time remaining, I want to write short stories about people I've known, like my aunt Shirley, married five times, and an actress in off-Broadway plays—vivacious isn't the word! In the stories I'd like to explore how the concept of time becomes so much more important as we age. I believe every one of us has stories inside that we need to share. Writing them down helps us understand ourselves and those we're close to.

Q: What effect does religious or spiritual practice have on your work?

A: With new patients I like to find out how faith affects their lives. Religious beliefs can offer tremendous support toward solving emotional problems. Faith is often a factor in deterring a patient from carrying out suicidal plans.

I myself am agnostic. Though raised in Judaism, I don't practice the rituals. I have lots of misgivings about the role that organized religion has played in crimes against humanity. In the eleventh, twelfth, and thirteenth centuries, the Crusaders forced other religious and cultural groups to convert to Catholicism or be punished. In the Middle East terrorists have distorted the values of Islam to justify bombings and beheadings.

The experience I've acquired from forty years of working with patients, plus surviving into my seventies, is largely what I fall back on to guide me in helping patients recover.

Q: What doubts and disappointments do you deal with in your work?

A: I get feelings of satisfaction when my efforts have had a positive effect on a person's life. When the opposite occurs, I ask myself, Is there anything I could have done differently to ameliorate the lives of those whose emotional problems overwhelm them?

Once in a while, self-destructive behavior is hard to mitigate. It's very sad. A thirty-eight-year-old, high-tech executive—who for several years had been trying to ease ongoing depression with alcohol—came to me. He'd been getting promotions regularly and, during our weekly visits, I encouraged him to explore becoming more involved with a woman he liked. The Prozac I prescribed seemed to be helping him a lot. He started attending AA meetings.

Then, suddenly, he had a reversal, missing two appointments in a row. I called his parents—neither they nor his employer knew where he was. Three weeks later, he phoned one morning, drunk, from a hotel in Albuquerque, whose name he didn't know. He agreed to call 911 because he'd fractured his wrist while in a drunken stupor.

Subsequently, I found out from his parents that he'd not called 911, that he'd drifted from motel to motel. No beds had been available in the hospital at the University of New Mexico, where his parents and I had wanted to take him. Several days afterward they managed to get him into a psychiatric hospital.

I haven't heard from them or him since. My guess is that the woman he liked, who was raising a little boy, had precipitated his relapse by refusing to embark on a life with him.

Q: How about an example of success?

A: A colleague referred a forty-three-year-old woman to me. She suffered from bipolar disorder: episodic depressions, apathy, social isolation, and lack of productivity in her career as a sculptor. For four years I saw her twice a month while carefully prescribing Lamictal for bipolar disorder, bupropion for depression, and Ritalin as an antidepressant booster.

The regular psychotherapeutic sessions, coupled with the medications, helped her recover from an ugly divorce, resume her career, and become engaged to a bank vice president who soon was promoted to president, necessitating a move to Denver. Before that happened, she was able to reduce her meds.

Q: **Will you share with readers what professional techniques you've come to trust?**

A: Sure. I convey empathy with the problems a patient faces, which helps establish and maintain a positive therapeutic relationship.

I spend a lot of time getting a thorough life history from the patient. I work hard to establish a trusting alliance. If pertinent, I try to figure out what factors are interfering with the patient's progress. What's contributing to the resistance to getting well? With the patient's permission, I like to confer—by phone, email, or visit—with her or his physician, social worker if any, family, and others important in the patient's life. As best I can, I individualize the treatment that seems best suited to the particular patient. I try to identify, and explain, major reasons that are stopping a patient from enjoying a more satisfying life.

Since medications have gotten far more sophisticated than they were even ten years ago, I take special care in choosing what's appropriate to each patient, begin with low doses to minimize side effects, and keep a close eye on how each patient is responding over time.

Lawrence Lazarus's Thumbnail Bio:

Born in Brooklyn, New York, 1941. BA, English, University of Pennsylvania, 1963. MD from Drexel Medical College, Pennsylvania, 1967. Residency in Psychiatry, Michael Reese Hospital, Chicago, 1968–1971. Assistant Professor of Psychiatry at Rush Medical College in Chicago, and Director, Geriatric Psychiatry Fellowship Program, 1977–2000. Private practice in Santa Fe, 2003–present. Founding member, American Association for Geriatric Psychiatry (AAGP), 1980; president, AAGP, 1988-1989. Coeditor, *Comprehensive Review of Geriatric Psychiatry*, American Psychiatric Press, 1996. Reviewer, *American Journal of Psychiatry*, 1978-1997. Psychiatric Consultant to La Familia Medical Center, 2010-2012. Author of book, *Getting the Health Care You Deserve in America's Broken Health Care System*, 2013.

Statistics on Mental Illness:

The World Health Organization (WHO) estimates that at least 25% of individuals worldwide develop one or more mental disorders. Most common are depression (10.4%) and generalized anxiety disorder (7.9%). Women are almost twice as likely to develop depression as men. The cost and emotional burden on families who care for people with severe mental problems is much higher than on those who care for people with chronic physical problems.

Suicide is among the ten leading causes of death for all ages in most countries.

The National Institute of Mental Health's *Epidemiologic Catchment Area Study* finds that in this country, the most common mental disorders for people over sixty-five are dementia, depression, phobias, and alcoholism. If diagnosed accurately, and treated in a timely manner, mild-to-moderate dementia can be slowed by administering a cholinesterase inhibitor such as Donepezil. Patients and their families can also benefit from psychotherapy.

To Learn More or Get Help:

National

    American Psychiatric Association
    1000 Wilson Blvd. Suite 1825   (continued)

Arlington, VA 22209-3901
(888) 357-7924
www.psychiatry.org

American Association for Geriatric Psychiatry
6728 Old McLean Village Drive
McLean VA, 22101-3906
(703) 556-9222
www.aagponline.org

In Santa Fe

Agavé Health, Inc
2504 Camino Entrada
Santa Fe, NM 87507-4851
(505) 471-5006
www.agavehealth.org

Christus St. Vincent Adult Behavioral Health Services
455 St. Michaels Drive
Santa Fe, NM 87505-7601
(505) 913-5470
www.stvin.org

Community Guidance Center
2960 Rodeo Park Drive West
Santa Fe, NM 87505-6351
(505) 986-9633
www.pmsnm.org

La Familia Medical Center
1035 Alto Street
Santa Fe, NM 87501-2406
(505) 982-4425
www.lafamiliasf.org

Cheryl Brown
Suicide-Loss Survivor, Psychotherapist

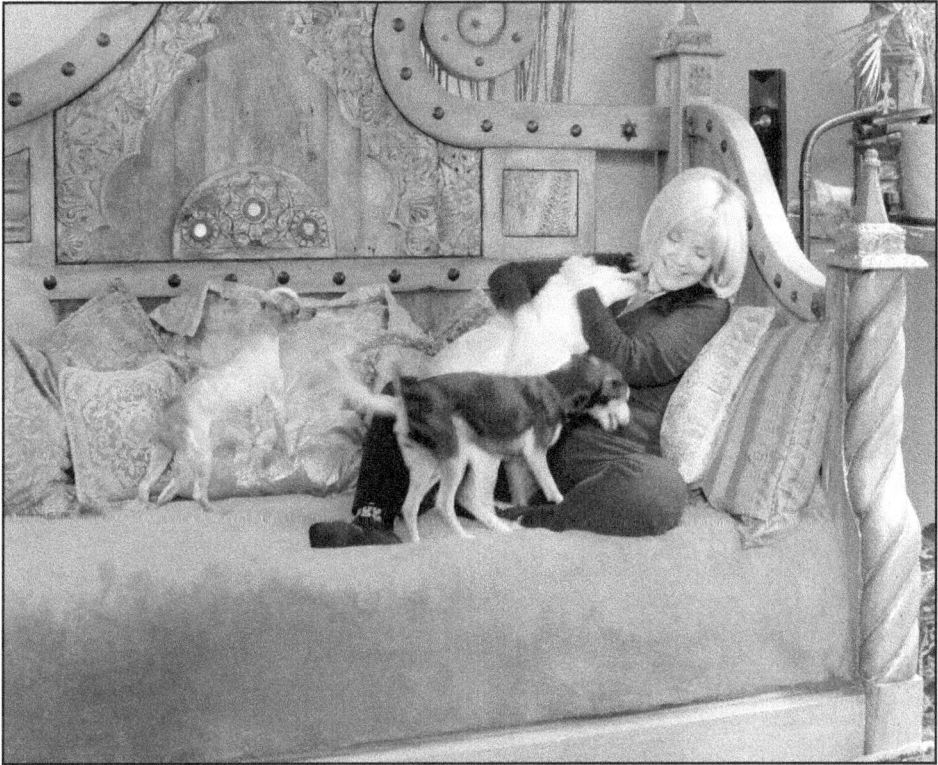

Q: Cheryl, tell us about your work with those left after a suicide.

A: Suicide-loss survivors need to be heard and understood. Why? We're nine times more likely to try suicide ourselves than the general public, which has placed a stigma on the subject.

In 1983, my estranged husband jumped off a cliff in Weisbaden, Germany. In 1989, I stopped drinking. In 2010, my son shot himself in Boulder, Colorado. I decided I could return to the bottle or live for my highest self by helping others voice their emotions, thoughts, and remembrances—without feeling judged. So I built two websites and a presence on Facebook. It took three months of planning and nine months of research and development. I worked twelve hours a day.

SuicideFindingHope.com has two hundred pages, attracting suicide-loss families and friends from all over the world. It's where I learned what PTSD (post-traumatic stress disorder) is doing to our soldiers returning from Iraq and Afghanistan. They're haunted by visions of death—an IED (improvised explosive device) detonating, a couple of buddies lying injured, one with his leg blown off. These veterans start panicking, avoiding people, refusing to drive because a car might backfire, a passenger door might slam. They become hypervigilant. Handguns are the most common way veterans kill themselves, having been trained in the armed services to use a Beretta M9 pistol or, earlier, a Colt 1911. In America, fifty percent of all suicides are by guns, seventy-five percent in the South.

People who suicide don't really want to die. They want to escape their pain and can't think of any other way to do it. They've often tried antidepressants, antipsychotics, tranquilizers. They consider themselves a burden on their families, having come to believe the world would be a better place without them. *SuicideFindingHope.com* shows them they're not alone, that their feelings are common. Millions of other sufferers will understand because they're going through the same thing. Viewers of this website can write in, telling their stories.

On *Facebook.com/SuicideFindingHope*, I post a thought and wait for responses. I posted about the copilot on a Germanwings jet, an offshoot of Lufthansa, who flew one-hundred-and-fifty passengers into a French Alp, killing everyone. The copilot's parents told reporters, "We noticed nothing wrong." My post asked Facebook viewers, "Do you think a suicidal person can hide his or her intensions?" Of course! It's easy to do.

SantaFeSurvivorsOfSuicide.com automatically gets whatever I post on Facebook. The home page reads, *We welcome all persons affected by the suicide of another person to our support group that meets the first and third*

Thursday of each month from 5:15 to 6:45 in the library of the Unitarian Universalist Church. Participation is free of charge.

In this group, death by handgun or hanging are common topics—one out of five sufferers from bipolar disorder attempt to take their lives like this, especially when they're flipping from mania to depression. I recall a couple of parents telling about their bipolar daughter—in grad school at Columbia—coming home for the holidays. They asked her to join them for dinner out. She refused, saying she needed to rest. Later they found her hanging by a scarf from the chandelier in her bedroom. She'd kicked the chair out from under her. Two days before, the psychiatrist at a hospital had reassured the parents, concerned about her moods, that she was not suicidal.

This couple attended our group for nearly three years. The first year they couldn't talk about much of anything without breaking into weeping. "Hang in there," someone thoughtlessly said, and the mother started bawling. Her husband took down the light fixture. Both avoided the room, wanting to sell the house but deciding they couldn't afford it. They told us that every morning, on waking up, they relived the experience, and feared going crazy. The PTSD-incited panic attacks felt like someone smashing a fist into their chests.

My own days are quite routine. I get up at six, brew a cup of coffee, eat a protein bar, and after talking on the phone a while with a friend, go into my library/office. There I enter Dante's lowest level of Hell, breathing in the pain of others to exhale hope. For two to four hours, seven days a week, I surf through Facebook and my two websites, reading stories, culling out anything too traumatic—like actual suicide notes—then post what's left by hitting the *Approve* button.

In 2013, I was diagnosed with CLL (Chronic Lymphocytic Leukemia), which I'm going to beat, though few have, with a couple dozen supplements, a few meds, and twelve varieties of teas. Plus, I eat carefully: string cheese, nuts and raisins for lunch, a bowl of blueberries and kefir for dinner, topped by broken walnuts—fine dining, according to me.

Two afternoons a week I volunteer in the chemotherapy room at

Christus St. Vincent's Cancer Center, disinfecting the chairs, bringing pillows, warmed blankets, and snacks to patients and trying to be a good listener. Emotional suffering is worse than physical suffering; the room is fear-based, though love permeates everything. Another afternoon I sort groceries that supermarkets donate to Food Depot, organizing deliveries to a hundred and fifty agencies in northern New Mexico. When I have the energy, I help out at annual charities like the International Folk Art Market in July and Indian Market in August. And I try to attend Santa Fe Survivors of Suicide sessions at the church every other Thursday evening.

When time allows, I call on pastors and priests—as well as the directors of Santa Fe's funeral homes—to assist development of appropriate religious or memorial services for people left behind after a suicide. And I'm helping several support groups expand this work into Albuquerque and elsewhere.

Q: Please expand on the life experiences that have contributed to your doing this good work.

A: I was raised in Oil City, Pennsylvania, fifteen thousand people who lived together in mutual trust. At age twenty-six I married a brilliant, troubled man five years older than me, believing if I loved him enough, he'd heal. The truth? I never really loved him. We became codependent, having met in Detroit, where I was teaching English and art at Salina Junior High. Gordon was chief designer for Pontiac, the youngest chief designer General Motors had ever had.

At the time I was also working toward my PhD in psychology at the University of Michigan, an hour's drive away. For a statistics class we asked friends to take an IQ test. The top possible score was 165. Gordon exceeded that. His intelligence allowed him to create a persona of normalcy.

In 1983 we'd been married eleven years and Gordon had become Director of Design for GM in Europe. We were living in Weisbaden, Germany. He had grown abusive. I'm five foot three, he was six foot four.

Blaming and screaming had progressed to hitting, first me, then our four-year-old son. Eric and I left Germany to go live with my parents in Oil City. I refused to consider reconciling until my husband sought psychiatric help. The doctor diagnosed him as bipolar but he refused treatment, fearing GM would fire him. A couple of months after I filed for divorce, he jumped off a cliff locals called "suicide mountain," overlooking the Rhine.

There was, still is, such shame associated with suicide that GM covered it up, producing a press release that claimed Gordon had stumbled while taking photos on a bird-watching tour and slipped to his death. He never watched birds! Me a blonde and him with reddish mustache and trimmed beard, for years we'd been the handsome couple with happy faces that went to all the cocktail parties. Looking back, I feel such a fraud.

Two days before Gordon died he called me from Weisbaden, asking for one last chance. I said no. The next night he phoned his brother here in the States, saying he was going to kill himself. He'd threatened that before; so often suicides are the boys who cry wolf. His brother didn't take him seriously.

Do I blame myself for Gordon's death? I used to, one hundred percent. "If only I had gone back to him," I thought. Researchers have identified a possible gene that causes bipolar disorder. It's probably inheritable. After we married, he told me his mother had suicided by overdosing on prescription drugs. He refused to talk about it ever again. And later, Eric, during his own manic rages, blamed me for marrying his father, which, of course, I internalized. Now, however, I don't blame myself at all. This is simply the path my life has taken and it's taught me so much. I no longer believe in blame. I try not to judge.

I was thirty-seven and Eric was five when Gordon died. We moved back to Detroit, where I resumed teaching art and later doing post-masters work in alcohol and drug abuse counseling at Wayne State University.

We left Detroit in 1986 for Kansas City to be nearer my older sister, so that if anything happened to me, she could care for Eric. I made my living as a therapist for multiple-DUI (Driving Under the Influence) offenders. I had used alcohol to push down all the feelings surrounding my husband's death—German beer was my drink of choice—but sobered up three years later, a few years before Eric, at fifteen, was diagnosed with his father's disease. It had been my greatest fear. Eric's mood swings and bouts of anger often devolved into severe depression, even though he stayed in therapy once a week, and trying to fix him became my full-time job. I was terrified, frustrated, and grew completely codependent.

Eric managed to graduate from the University of Kansas with a BS in Exercise Physiology in 2002. He became a personal trainer in Boulder and I moved to Santa Fe, where I'd always loved the architecture and terrain. I retired as a therapist but volunteered to give behavioral tests to the dogs coming into the county's animal shelter.

A good-looking kid who often told me he felt ugly, Eric took his life in June, 2010. He left behind lots of girlfriends who had bowed out after nine to twelve months, tiring of his mood swings. A few still write me on his angelversary, the date of his death.

A month before he died, Eric snail-mailed me a letter. "Mom," he wrote, "there's something wrong with my brain. I've known it for a long time and I don't know what to do."

In Boulder he got into organic foods, associated with people living a natural lifestyle—during the autopsy, the coroner found a salad in his stomach. He'd quit therapy, stopped the Lamictal for his bipolar disorder, refused to try Zoloft because it dampened his libido.

Eric's computer had crashed; on the day he died he brought home a new one from Best Buy to assemble. Earlier he'd purchased a used Glock 17 pistol, claiming an increase in neighborhood robberies. Five months before, at Christmas, I'd made him promise that he'd never use the gun on himself.

The coroner and police did a psychological autopsy—it's becoming a big thing with suicides. Judging by the helter-skelter positions of the new-computer cartons and components, they figured Eric had had a meltdown, then went into the closet where he kept the gun. So that blood wouldn't make a mess on the floor, Eric had laid his head sideways in the gun case and squeezed the trigger.

Q: Any current role models who inspire you?

A: Every human being is a role model. Each has something to teach, and for that I am grateful. You're my hero today. If I had a choice between lunch with you and Noreen (the interviewer's late wife) and the Dalai Lama, I wouldn't care whom. I've learned not to put anyone on a pedestal.

Some of my greatest teachers have been those who've pissed me off the most. That way I've learned whom I don't want to emulate.

I was once volunteering in the chemotherapy room, attending a Hispanic gentleman with stage-four cancer. That's as bad as it gets, spread everywhere, usually incurable. I brought a pillow, put a heated blanket around his shoulders, served him snacks and tea. A slight man in his seventies, head still full of shining black hair, he wore a pressed shirt. Smiled nonstop, had smile wrinkles all over his face.

I told him how much I admired his attitude. He replied that his family thinks he's crazy, smiling and laughing so much when he's dying.

And there's a friend of mine, who, even though she's married, calls me every weekday morning to talk politics and share experiences about people we've encountered in the past twenty-four hours. We're on the phone for forty-five minutes. It's like a therapy session. We met years ago at the Santa Fe Animal Shelter. Afterward, at the computer in my den, I'm able to be more present and useful for the friends and relatives of suicides.

Q: How do you arrange the rest of your life to let you do this good work?

A: I'm not arranging the rest of my life. I live in the now, attending only to what's in front of me, this moment. That's all that exists. You know the saying, "Wherever you are, try to be there?" That's what I do.

Even when I'm not feeling well, and unable physically to be of use to others, I can breathe in others' suffering, transform it, and breathe out compassion.

Q: What effect does religious or spiritual practice have on your work?

A: Dogma and ritual are of no interest; what does interest me is my twelve-step program as it intertwines with Buddhist philosophy.

That philosophy says life is suffering. The greatest cause of suffering is attachment—to work, to liquor, to loving too much, to exercise, food, sex, gambling. When I need to find a way to detach from suffering, or arrive at any other decision, I imagine myself in a boat, heading towards certainty if I keep rowing every day. By rowing I mean helping to relieve the suffering of others as well as attending to the minutiae of life—dressing, flossing, washing the dishes, paying bills. If I do that, I believe a higher intelligence, as my rudder, will lead me to the right shore.

I have a strong belief in the soul, that part of us that never dies. For me it's a flower that transcends when the body's life is over. I call our present existence 'earth school'—we are here to learn. I try to turn each day into an ongoing prayer.

When I get up every morning, I do ask what I call The Source to be guided on how best to serve others.

Q: Any doubts or disappointments?

A: One Wednesday, dining with friends at Jambo Cafe, I ordered something that sounded tantalizing, highly spiced vegetable soup, even though I knew it wouldn't agree with me. It certainly didn't agree with me. Going for temporary pleasure in exchange for long-term discomfort is always unwise because I can't help others as I should. You know how physiologists call our stomach the second brain? It's been keeping me from making effective decisions.

After any negative experience, I ask, What can I learn from this?

In order to be useful, I have to keep my body healthy. And so I learn and move on. After all the crap I've gone through, I lead a wonderful life. I laugh a lot!

Q: Some examples of your successes helping others?

A: In general, I don't like the term 'success' because it's societally defined. Though I certainly consider my dogs from the shelter—the two Santa Fe blends, Chai and Roark, and ZuZu, my Mexican hairless—to be successes. Unlike theirs, my ego craves adulation; I'm trying to put it to rest. That said, here's a story. A few years ago, a woman's mother and would-have-been mother-in-law brought her kicking and screaming into our Survivors of Suicide meeting. In her mid-twenties, she possessed long black hair and a Masters in Sociology. Pain twisted her face, which otherwise was stunning. One evening her fiancé—a carpenter—and she, drinking bourbon, were making plans for their wedding in the living room of the home he had built for them. She wanted at least a hundred guests and elaborate flower arrangements. He told her, "Get over it, stop all this dreaming, we don't have the money." The bickering escalated. He stomped into the bedroom, returned with a handgun, and shot himself in the face.

Though heavily medicated when we met her, she kept shouting she also had to die, to be with him. I told her that night, and for months afterward, that she could look forward to an amazing future, just as I had found. She kept insisting that she'd never lose the visual of his bloody face. Not only was she furious with him, but felt one hundred percent responsible for his death.

Some time back I was in the legislators' chamber of the state capitol, to celebrate Survivors of Suicide Recognition Day. A senator's aide got up and rushed toward me. It was the woman I mentioned above. She gave me a huge hug, started crying out of gratitude that I'd presented her with hope when she'd had none.

Here's another story: A woman in her early sixties joined our group in 2012. She dressed conservatively—dark skirt, blouse, a string of pearls. Very articulate. She'd lived a long time in Tokyo, where her husband was chief financial officer for a multinational.

A month before we met, her younger brother—a dairyman in Wisconsin, much beloved as a volunteer fireman and city counselor—careful not to wake his wife, crawled out of bed after midnight, drove to the community water tower, climbed to the top, and jumped to his death. He left no explanatory note; only one in five suicides does. All he left were details about debts he owed a couple of banks.

His wife felt devastated. How could he take up so much paper describing what he wanted done with the farm, and no words of love for her?

His sister was equally traumatized, showing all the symptoms of PTSD: staring into space or hypervigilant, an exaggerated startle response. If someone in our group set down a coffee cup, and it clinked, she would jump. She insisted her life was over, blaming herself because she hadn't stayed in enough contact with her brother. When someone suicides, everyone who felt close tends to self-blame.

Early last year, she and I met for lunch and she shared that her life had blossomed. She'd put herself in therapy, and her marriage had grown happy again.

There's an equation I see working over and over: R equals E plus I. R is reality, E is the event, I is how the survivor interprets the event. After a lot of work, that interpretation can change from "My life is over; no one will ever forgive me" to "She or he made the choice; I now forgive her or him as well as myself."

Cheryl Brown's Thumbnail Bio:

Born in Oil City Pennsylvania, 1946. BA Humanities, University of New Mexico, 1968. MA Psychology, University of Michigan (U of M), 1972. One hundred twenty hours toward PhD in Psychology, U of M and Wayne State University. Taught junior high English and art, Arabic neighborhood in Dearborn, Michigan, for 17 years. Made health-care checks for Americans in German prisons, 1980-1983. Worked as psychotherapist with multiple-DUI offenders, most of whom were alcoholics, in Shawnee Mission, Kansas, 1990-2000. Created and services two websites and a presence on Facebook for families and friends of suicides, 2010-present.

Statistics on Suicide:

Each year, one million people worldwide take their own lives. Women make the attempt three times oftener than men. Ninety percent of suicides have suffered at least one episode of mental illness, mainly depression, itself the #1 disability in the world. Most depression is manageable, using therapy and medications.

In the United States, nearly 40,000 suicides occur annually, following a million tries. Four times as many men succeed as women. Of the two million Americans struggling with bipolar disorder, a fourth to a half make at least one attempt to end their lives; half of those use a firearm. More U.S. servicemen and women die by suicide than in combat; twenty-two U.S. veterans take their lives every day.

In Asia, the most common method of suicide is swallowing a pesticide.

To Learn More, or Get Help:

Cheryl Brown's Online Services
>SuicideFindingHope.com
>Facebook.com/SuicideFindingHope
>SantaFeSurvivorsOfSuicide.com

Other Services
>American Association for Suicidology
>5221 Wisconsin Ave. NW
>Washington, DC 20015   (continued)

(202) 237-2280
www.suicidology.org

American Foundation for Suicide Prevention
120 Wall Street, 29th Floor
New York, NY 10005
(212) 363-3500
Toll-Free: (888) 333-2377
www.afsp.org

The Link Counseling Center for Suicide Prevention and Aftercare
348 Mt. Vernon Hwy NE
Sandy Springs, GA 30328
(404) 256-9797
www.thelink.org

National Suicide Prevention Lifeline
(800) 273-8255

In Santa Fe

Santa Fe Survivors of Suicide
Unitarian Universalist Church
107 Barcelona (and Galisteo)
Santa Fe, NM 87505
5:15-6:45 pm, first and third Thursdays
www.SantaFeSurvivorsOfSuicide.com

Gerard's House of Santa Fe
(for children up to age 21)
3204 Mercantile Court
Santa Fe, NM 87507
(505) 424-1800
www.gerardshouse.org

New Mexico Crisis and Access Line
(855) 662-7474

Russell Baker
Executive Director, National Dance Institute
New Mexico

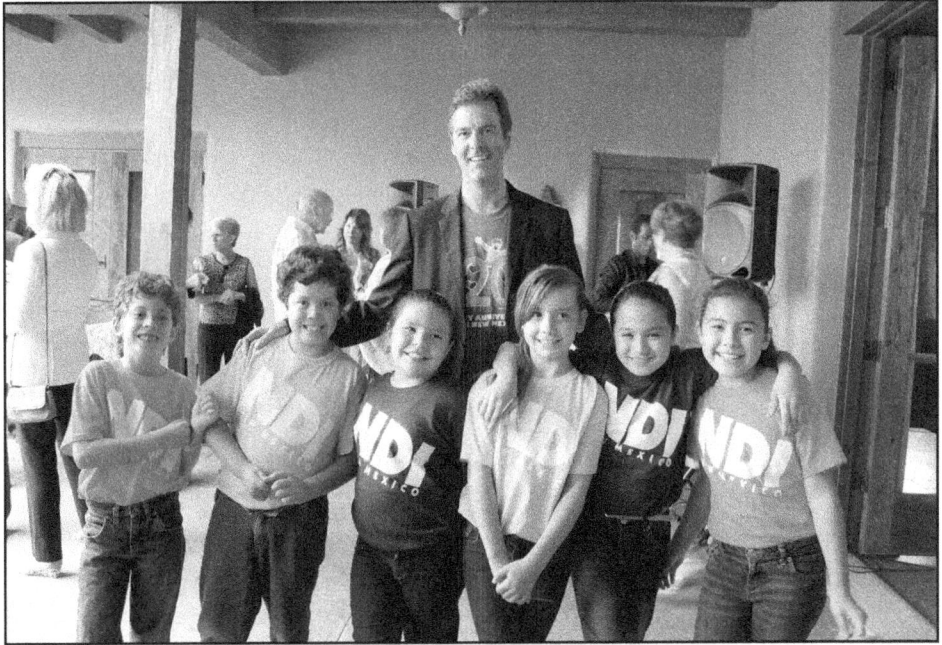

Q: Russell, what is the National Dance Institute (NDI) New Mexico all about?

A: NDI New Mexico is dedicated to using dance for inspiring elementary-school children to work hard, do their best, never give up, and stay healthy.

We serve nine thousand children at little or no cost in thirty-four communities and eighty-five schools. We work with entire classes, such as twenty-five fourth graders at El Camino Real Elementary in Santa Fe.

An NDI pianist and a dance teacher visit once a week for fifty minutes during the school year. Using the gym or cafeteria, they teach a fast-paced, high-energy, fun class involving call-and-response games, urging the kids toward their personal best.

The Music Game, for instance, goes like this: the pianist plays music evocative of, say, joy, and the children move accordingly. When the pianist stops, everyone freezes; those who don't are out. He starts up again, evoking a different emotion—say sorrow—and the children respond. They continue expressing emotions in this way for seven minutes or so.

Runs and Jumps starts with the children standing against the wall. The dance teacher has taped a big, colored X in the middle of the floor. As the pianist plays, each child runs to the X, jumps over it, stretches her or his arms overhead, and smiles toward where an audience might be sitting at their End-of-Year Event in May.

The kids also learn choreography; the dance teacher shows them how to break down a step. They may first practice a step's rhythm by clapping hands, then learn how to jump, next how to rotate the forearms around each other like rolling pins, then how to twist sideways while keeping their faces toward the front, and finally how to put it all together.

At the end of the school year, all our kids perform on stage in their communities—at The Dance Barns in Santa Fe, for instance, and at The Hiland Theater in Albuquerque. Those who have shown exceptional ability can join the Super Wonderful Advanced Team—we call it SWAT—and perform as well.

In Santa Fe and Albuquerque, any child of any age can attend classes after school, on Saturdays, and in the summer.

Q: Tell us what you do as Executive Director.

A: I started out in 2002 as an NDI dance teacher in Española, Chimayo, and Dulce. When I became Artistic Director of NDI New Mexico, I wrote scripts for our End-of-Year Events and trained other teachers.

All this experience helped when I became Executive Director, based in Santa Fe, in 2008.

The job brings many parts of my life together. Being an English major at Vassar instilled the importance of communicating ideas clearly, through writing and speaking, whether I'm talking to a board member, a donor, or a parent.

I started dancing late, as a sophomore at Vassar. Afterward, I performed for ten years with the Kansas City Ballet. From choreographing I learned how a teacher inspires performers to move in a way that expresses whatever feeling or idea you want to convey.

Mostly what I do now is try to communicate the vision and mission of NDI to fund-raisers, volunteers, public officials, business leaders, and the kids themselves.

New York City Ballet's Jacques d'Amboise founded NDI in 1976 from the conviction that the arts have a unique power to engage children. Our programs help them develop discipline, a standard of excellence, and a belief in themselves that carries over into all aspects of their lives. Often people get a misconception, because of the word *dance*, of what we're about. A few years ago we were having a hard time getting a community leader to come see a class, a demonstration, or a performance. He finally came to a board-member's home for what we call a 'cultivation event.' A pianist, a dance teacher, and a small group of children put on a mini-demonstration of our techniques. The man fell instantly in love, becoming a board member himself and one of our most ardent supporters.

I'd like to tell you about one student. She was studying to become a nurse practitioner as a grad student at the University of New Mexico. Growing up in Pojoaque just north of Santa Fe, she started with us in fourth grade. Like so many children in New Mexico, she didn't have a lot of exposure to opportunities such as NDI. Many of our public schools don't offer art or music programs, even physical education.

She went through Outreach, SWAT, and our Celebration Team. She took Dance Barn classes and became a member of Company XCel, a pre-professional group of our most advanced dancers. Her parents drove her to classes and Saturday rehearsals, and volunteered to usher, organize costumes, and chaperone.

While in grad school she worked as a nurse in the children's oncology unit at the University of New Mexico Hospital. She has told me she misses dancing, that she plans to take an NDI class at the Hiland Theater in Albuquerque. "NDI showed me that, if you work hard, anything is possible," she said. The impact of the program has made her want to help New Mexico children have better lives.

Q: What life experiences have contributed to your doing this good work?

A: My younger brother and I moved from Iowa to Minnesota, to Connecticut, and to Austin, Texas with caring parents. They instilled in us the values of commitment and integrity. We spent lots of time together— family dinners, vacations to Disney World, and to visit my grandparents and cousins in West Texas. My parents made sure we participated in sports like swimming and soccer and especially tennis.

From ages six to eight, I used to go to the Saturday art school for kids at the University of Minnesota. My mom taught art education at the university. I soaked up a lot about what it takes to be a good teacher.

I've also learned valuable life lessons through music. My grandmother had given our family a Baldwin upright piano. When I reached first grade I told my mom, "I'm ready to learn how to play this thing." She hired our school's music teacher to come to our house once a week. When I skipped practice, I had to fess up.

Piano lessons lead to recitals, which means playing from memory. I hated that because as soon as I had to look at the keys without a score, in front of all those parents, I couldn't remember a thing. But I didn't want to quit. So I convinced the teacher to let me use the score, even though no one else did. It's when I realized the power of the gift of persuasion.

In third grade I took up the clarinet. My dad had been drum major in his high school's band and played the instrument. I wanted to carry on some of the family tradition. So I played clarinet in my own high school's band and at Vassar in the orchestra, continuing piano on my own.

I recall once having to come back early to Poughkeepsie after winter break to rehearse a Brahms symphony, as well as my clarinet solo in Gershwin's *American in Paris*. It made me so proud to be working with all those people to present our best selves to an audience.

Performing for ten years with the Kansas City Ballet helped me become disciplined. Except for Sunday, every day I'd arrive at the studio an hour early to stretch and warm up. Class ran from nine to ten-thirty. Rehearsals started at eleven and often lasted until five-thirty. I'd have dinner, then take another class or work out at the gym. Since I didn't start dancing until later in life, I always felt I had to train and perform full out.

A professional company is continually working to stage a production. Our four performance seasons were October, December for the *Nutcracker*, February, and May. I learned how a large group of people go about coordinating choreography, music, costumes, dancing, lighting, sets, and props to present an artistic vision at the highest level.

Q: Any role models who inspire you?

A: Catherine Oppenheimer, our founding Artistic Director, started NDI New Mexico in 1994, after she had danced for Balanchine at New York City Ballet, and worked with Jacques d'Amboise at NDI New York. She has long blonde hair, often worn in a ponytail. You never know when she's going to break into dance. When she looks at you, you feel like the most important person in the world. With all her grace, Catherine also has a lot of what she calls testosterone. She's galvanized so many of us; she's a visionary with an endless well of energy. She has a vision to lead the drive to build a permanent home for the New Mexico School for the Arts, a statewide, public, residential high school for the performing and visual arts.

The other role models I'm inspired by are the many philanthropists effecting positive change in our communities and the world. The late

Don Chalmers, who owned Don Chalmers Ford, was one of these. A big man with a heart to match, he helped bring people together around good ideas like renovating the Hiland Theater in Albuquerque for NDI New Mexico.

Q: How do you arrange the rest of your life to let you do this good work?

A: When you're doing what I am, you don't take a lot of time off. I've got a friend who asks, "Are we ever going to play tennis?" I say, "I'll let you know when," but I never have time, so she never hears from me.

I wake at six and work for a couple of hours on my laptop. As soon as I get to The Dance Barns, it's meetings or responding to the needs of different people in different departments—our New Mexico staff has grown to a hundred. Plus I spend as much time as possible with donors.

My partner and I have been together for twenty-three years. I get home about the same time he does. I'll fix dinner or we'll go out, and then I'm back on my laptop for another hour or two. Saturdays I'm at the Barns for six hours, choreographing and trying to help the other teachers strengthen their relationships with students.

Because of the grueling hours, I'm attempting to rearrange my work life, not burn out. Staff and I are talking about how I can delegate more, whom we can put into leadership positions.

On Sundays I like to ride my bike or hike. The mind can wander or just be quiet.

When I moved out to New Mexico in 2002, I thought I'd have a lot of free time to be a writer, a dream that started at Vassar. I had this vision that New Mexico's big night sky so full of stars represented what I could do as a writer. In college I wrote poetry; now I'd like to try a screenplay or a novel.

Q: What effect does religious or spiritual practice have on your work?

A: No current practice but a lesson from the past helps:

For a long time my brother and I refused to go to church. "What if you could choose, would you go?" my parents asked. "Yes," we said. We were living outside of Minneapolis, and spent a year sampling all sorts of denominations, finally choosing the Lutheran church because of the guitarist and the singing. The pastor was an inspiration. He had the kids sit by the altar for a special children's sermon. It seemed like he had dedicated his life to the congregation, helping us find our rightful place in the world. The stories in his sermons ended as life lessons for me, like do unto others as you would have them do unto you, and be there for people less fortunate.

Before we left Minnesota for Connecticut—I was in third grade— the pastor was in a car accident, and fell into a coma. My parents tried to explain but I couldn't understand where this person I loved had gone.

In Connecticut the strangest thing happened. We had joined another Lutheran church. A few years later, I picked up the church bulletin, which I wasn't in the habit of doing, and read that the pastor who meant so much to me, who'd never awakened, had died. It saddened me deeply. There had been a person who'd made a difference in my life simply by being himself. Well, I thought, isn't that the greatest thing you can do?

Q: What doubts and disappointments do you deal with in your work?

A: Mostly what keeps me up at night is worrying that we won't be able to secure the funds needed to sustain what's become a large and complicated operation. Complications include finding enough teachers who have the skills, high energy, and upbeat spirit to carry out the program. New Mexico does not appeal to everyone. If you're a principal dancer in New York, moving west to teach dance in a cafeteria in Alamogordo to kids who don't yet know their right from their left, let alone how to count to eight, may not be on your radar. Dancers who are done performing have to love it here, the slower pace, no city-life buzz. But sometimes Santa Fe can feel isolating, hard to find a network of friends.

Training a dancer to teach the NDI program takes from one to two years. A big disappointment is having that person think soon after, I've had my New Mexico experience, time to move on. You have to have some kind of connection, perhaps a relative who lives nearby, happy memories from childhood, *something*, in order to last. So often those who come out only for adventure, one day want to go back to their lives.

How to maintain the quality of our programs and performances are two of my concerns. When we had just a handful of teachers, we could have a more relaxed environment. The bigger we've become, the more classrooms there are to visit, the more relationships to manage with staff and donors, the more to keep in balance. Today we're following more policies than ever, more systems.

This year we're doing great, serving a lot of kids. The expectation is that next year we'll do even better. Can we live up to this?

Sure, sometimes we stumble. A performance where the kids aren't ready becomes stressful for everyone. So does a fund-raiser where a donor's badge is missing or a name's not on the guest list. To a child, the dance teacher who leaves halfway through a school year is the most stressful event of all.

Q: A couple more examples of your successes?

A: The greatest sense of accomplishment happens when a former student, breaking into a smile, walks up to one of us to say what they're doing now and recalls how important NDI New Mexico has been, the friendships made. In Santa Fe this happens often, in a restaurant, a bank, a grocery store.

Just last month the Stephan Petronio Dance Company in New York hired one of our students as a member. As a youngster she had struggled with reading. But in fourth grade at Pojoaque Elementary, she discovered her passion for dancing. She applied the NDI principals of work hard, never give up, do your best, and moved up through SWAT, our Celebration Team, and Company XCel until graduating at eighteen. She studied at Point Park University in Pittsburgh, then moved to New York

City where she auditioned and studied dance for four to five years until last month's offer came from the Stephan Petronio group.

I remember her with her brown hair in a bun and pretty dark eyes getting the lead in our End-of-Year Event, *Joe Kid for President*. Having just signed a mock bill into law, she stood on stage, on a desk under a huge crayon, and shouted, "I did it!"

Another student, like a lot of our kids, loved playing football, and didn't seem like he was going to stick with dance. At times he seemed like the best dancer out there, at times he seemed uninterested. In seventh grade, he injured his ankle. This is it, we thought; we've lost him. But we were wrong. He had a growth spurt and got back into dancing. You could see in how he moved that he was discovering a new strength and expressiveness. He recognized that all of us saw that something special was happening. He came to the Dance Barns every day, stretching and doing strengthening exercises in a corner, taking classes, watching the older dancers perform.

Most days, back then, after fixing breakfast for his mom when she wasn't well enough to drive, he took the bus or walked the mile from home. At fourteen years old, still mischievious but no longer so small, Terrance graduated from Celebration Team to join Company XCel.

Q: How do you go about fund-raising?

A: We try to leave no stone unturned, reaching out to individuals, businesses, foundations, and government. We create earned-income opportunities like videos and raffle tickets, as well as solicit advertisements in our program books.

At five hundred dollars a couple, our number one fund raiser is the Gala, held when the school year ends. After the students perform on stage, they line up, each holding a balloon, to guide guests toward a white tent set up in the parking lot. From the kids you hear a lot of "Thanks for coming to the show," and "Thanks for supporting us," plus comments like,

"I love your earrings." Buses return them to their schools, where parents pick them up.

Guests dress up for the Gala, men in suits, women in cocktail dresses. They enter the tent a little before seven, are served dinner and entertained by a band. The high spirits of the children pervade the evening, ending at nine-thirty. A photographer takes color shots of every guest, which we mail out later. Raffle prizes are awarded, Company XCel performs, and then I walk onto the portable floor to say, "Okay, we all know there's one more thing to do." I ask everyone willing to pledge a thousand dollars for sponsoring one child for a year, to come up beside me.

It's important to cultivate a broad base of support from donors who give less than a thousand a year. To those who join our Founders Circle by offering more, we offer special benefits: preferred seating and a cocktail party, plus reserved parking and attendance at a master's class.

Those giving at least ten thousand dollars to sponsor a class at one of our elementary schools belong to our Circle of Excellence.

All donors of five hundred dollars and more receive a thank-you from one of our children—a handwritten letter or card, a drawing or other artwork.

The Silver Sneakers Legacy Society's benefactors have included NDI New Mexico in their estate planning. We ask those most passionate about our mission to join. All have a silver sneaker, hand-painted with their name, added to the mobile in our lobby.

Now I'll tell you what *doesn't* work—mistakes like misspelling a donor's name or leaving it off a donor-recognition list. The level of upset rises as the money given rises. You feel terrible when it happens.

Not saying thank you in a timely manner is another mistake. So is asking for too little. Some donors will be offended if you don't ask for enough.

Let's say someone has just given ten thousand dollars. We better not request another thousand two months later, though we may ask if the patron would be willing to host a dinner party.

Russell Baker's Thumbnail Bio:

Born in Ames, Iowa, 1968. Started dancing in 1988 at Vassar College; earned BA in English there, 1991. MFA Ballet Teaching and Choreography, University of Utah, 1994. Danced with Kansas City Ballet, 1993–2003. Founded Kansas City Contemporary Dance Ensemble, 1999. Kansas City Ballet performed Baker's *The Cloud Chamber* in 2002. Directed National Dance Institute's (NDI's) North and Santa Fe programs, 2002–2004. Became NDI New Mexico's Artistic Director in 2004 and Executive Director in 2008.

Statistics re: the National Dance Institute (NDI):

NDI New Mexico was founded in 1994. Its staff of 100 serves 9,000 public elementary school children, their 700 teachers, and 75,000 audience members in thirty-four urban, rural, and Native American communities. Life lessons it teaches through the arts have resulted in grade-point averages 30-42% higher than the averages of nonparticipants. Sixty-five-percent of participants are Hispanic, 20% Anglo, 12% Native American, 2% African American, 1% Asian.

NDI itself was founded in 1976 by New York City Ballet principal dancer Jacques d'Amboise. Associates of National Dance Institute (ANDI) include arts-education organizations serving low-income families in ten other states.

To Learn More or Get Involved:

National Dance Institute (NDI) New Mexico
    1140 Alto Street
    Santa Fe, NM 87501
    (505) 983-7646
    www.ndi-nm.org

National Dance Institute (NDI)
    217 W. 147th Street
    New York, NY 10039
    (212) 226-0083
    www.nationaldance.org

Associates of National Dance Institute (ANDI)

California
California Dance Institute
The Capshaw-Spielberg Center
3131 Olympic Blvd, Suite 202
Santa Monica, CA 90404
(323) 301-8900
www.californiadanceinstitute.org

Colorado
Celebrate the Beat
PO Box 1974
Aspen, CO 81612
(970) 433-2585
www.ctbeat.org

Idaho
Treasure Valley Institute for Children's Arts
1406 Eastman Street
Boise, ID 83702
(208) 703-5615
www.trica.org

Illinois
Chicago Dance Institute
1800 N. Hermitage
Chicago, IL 60622
(773) 698-6475
www.chicagodanceinstitute.org

New Hampshire
New Hampshire Dance Institute
PO Box 1116
Keene, NH 03431
(603) 355-8911
www.nhdi.org

New Jersey

Trenton Education Dance Institute
c/o Children's Home Society
635 S. Clinton Avenue
Trenton, NJ 08611
(609) 695-6274
www.chsofnj.org

North Carolina

Arts in Action
PO Box 51277
Durham, NC 27717
(919) 619-0483
www.ncartsinaction.org

Ohio

Momentum
PO Box 21224
Columbus, OH 43212
(614) 314-8251
www.momentum-excellence.org

Texas

Kids Excel
PO Box 920144
El Paso, TX 79902
(915) 351-6999
www.kids-excel.org

Virginia

Minds in Motion
Richmond Ballet
407 East Canal Street
Richmond, VA 23220
(804)344-0906
www.rbmim.com

Deborah Tang
Executive Director, St. Elizabeth Shelter

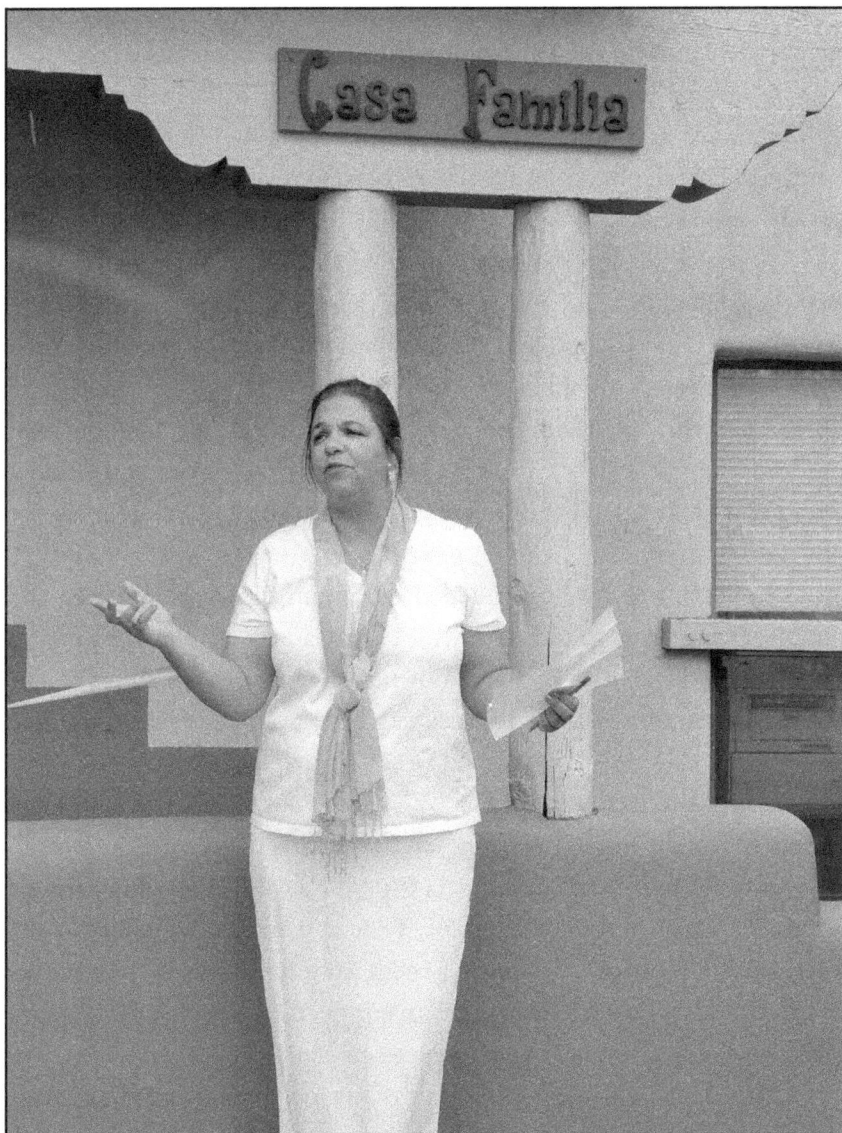

Q: Deborah, tell us about St. Elizabeth Shelter and your duties there.

A: Today, seventy-five percent of Americans are one or two paychecks away from homelessness. In New Mexico, at least seventeen thousand are homeless over the course of a year. St. Elizabeth serves a couple thousand of these in Santa Fe with two emergency shelters, three longer-term, supportive-housing complexes, a legal clinic, and a homeless court.

Our goal is to get as many as possible out of homelessness and into our units and others scattered around the city. My job is to carry out the will of the Board of Directors by building a can-do spirit among twenty-seven staff.

A few years ago the Board decided that if our men guests show that they're looking for a job or housing, applying for disability benefits, trying to reconnect with family, following doctor's orders regarding their meds—in other words, taking positive steps toward stable housing—we'll let them stay in the Men's Emergency Shelter for longer than our past maximum of thirty days. This is also true for single women and families with children at Casa Familia. We don't like to accept people if they're just passing through.

In 2012, when we open-ended maximum stays, two hundred and ninety-seven guests found housing. A year later, that number grew to three hundred and ninety, a thirty-one percent gain. Best of all, we're now able, before a month passes, to place nearly half our guests in permanent housing.

We like to have a variety of expertise on our Board. Currently that includes, among others, two lawyers, two formerly homeless women who had used our services, a media expert, a health-care administrator, a retired human-resources executive, a social worker, a book editor, and a retired Navajo Nation leader. We meet from five to seven-thirty every fourth Tuesday. Besides making all major decisions, they have the final say in resolving grievances among guests or staff.

Board relations are just one part of my job. Supporting our managers is another. Not only do I attend their case-management and monthly meetings, but am available 24/7 if they have a concern. We house guests, for instance, who act out behavioral-health issues. When a manager can't decide whether to call an ambulance, evict, or simply separate them from other guests, I'll get a call.

We had a man in our eight-unit senior apartments who owned a Rottweiler. Mostly passive, though occasionally it growled. Though it hadn't bit anyone, the other men and women felt threatened. The dilemma that the manager presented me was how to ensure the safety of everyone without taking away the man's right to a companion. Three other guests had dogs, but the situation got to be seven guests against one.

I called a meeting to lessen their fears. Then, after the manager and I met with each of the eight individually, we assembled again, and set a couple of rules. One, the man had to keep the dog on a leash when outside his apartment. Two, he and his dog had to back away from any guest who made that request.

Besides specially called get-togethers, staff and I meet for three hours, including lunch, once a month at the Men's Emergency Shelter, October through April. In warmer weather we rotate among the five facilities to help staff feel connected by better understanding how each program operates.

First we build community over lunch. The next hour is spent learning about a different Santa Fe nonprofit, or maybe CPR (cardiopulmonary resuscitation) training, or how to use a fire extinguisher, or how to maintain personal safety. Reports from each housing manager, our business manager, our development manager, and from me fill the rest of the afternoon.

The whole point of these meetings is to create cohesion; team-building is something we work on all the time. When I came on board nine years ago after supervising domestic-violence shelters in Farmington and Rio Rancho, each program at St. Elizabeth felt isolated. The managers seemed to be doing their own thing in their own corner of the universe.

Another part of my job is to cement good relations with local nonprofits connected to the work we do here. St. Elizabeth cooperates with the New Mexico Coalition to End Homelessness, the Tri-County Behavioral-Health Collaborative, the Salvation Army, Healthcare for the Homeless, Kitchen Angels, the Food Depot, the Esperanza Shelter for Battered Families, Planned Parenthood, Su Vida, Santa Fe Boys and Girls Club, and many more. Thus I may be going to a hospital meeting or a law-enforcement meeting or a behavioral-health meeting. It's of utmost importance to reduce duplication of services while also filling gaps—never losing sight of our mutual goal to stamp out homelessness.

I spend a lot of time talking to active and potential donors, giving tours of our facilities, and attending events. One of the biggest events is the Thornburg Investments/Wells Fargo Bank holiday party. There's tons of food—enchiladas, roast beef, side dishes, multiple desserts. At Casa Familia and Sonrisa, we house up to fifty children. Two months prior, they make out a wish list. Thornburg and Wells Fargo employees buy trikes, bikes, video games, clothes, shoes, and other gifts. Parents, kids, and staff then gather at the Dance Barns a week before Christmas to enjoy face-painting, Santa Claus, unicyclists, and mimes.

You can see that I wear many hats. As head honcho, sometimes I have to be the bad guy, the mediator. But I'm responsible for everything—the final say on data produced, job evaluations, expenditures, the approval of time cards. I sign all the checks, and send out thanks for monetary and other donations, like the turkeys and fixings LANL (Los Alamos National Labs) gives us every Thanksgiving.

Q: What life experiences have contributed to your doing this good work?

A: I was in an abusive marriage for ten years and my husband had threatened me if I ran away. But finally I did run, barefoot in December in Minneapolis in the snow. It was five miles to the hospital and I was thirty years old. The nurses wrapped me in blankets. Ninety percent of my body was covered with bruises from the beatings.

The next day I took the bus to get my ten-month-old son, Rahman, my two-year-old daughter, Josephine, and my six-year-old daughter, Ayanna. I'd forgotten to grab my purse from the house. But the bus driver took one look at my face and let us ride free to the domestic-violence shelter the nurses had told me about.

I'd been able to keep my job, working first in accounting, and later on the swing shift in the factory, doing quality assurance on circuit boards; the company manufactured computers. After four months at the shelter, I found housing. But my husband had someone follow me home from work, and he called that night to say he knew where the kids and I lived. So we returned to the shelter. The case manager found us a shelter in Denver. I drove the kids west and in a little time found a place to rent. The problem was that my paycheck did not cover expenses. Day care alone for three kids cost a hundred and fifty dollars a week. So off and on for nearly four years we were homeless, sleeping in parking lots in the van I'd bought. Whenever I accumulated enough money, we rented again.

After my husband died from complications due to alcoholism, and my kids were too old for day care, a friend in Eugene, Oregon, said we could stay with her. At the age of thirty-eight I was accepted at Oregon State there. I found part-time work doing accounting at a halfway house for people coming out of the state's mental institution, until I'd earned my BA in Political Science. Four years later, I received two masters' degrees from the University of New Mexico, in Community and Regional Planning and in Latin American Studies.

When I started ten years after that at St. Elizabeth's, I wanted to offer a safe place for women and children, in addition to our existing facility for men. The rule with domestic-violence shelters is that the woman must be in 'immediate danger' to stay. Once you leave, you can't return unless you're again in immediate danger. There is no such rule at our Casa Familia—for women with children and for women alone—that opened in 2005, four years after I came on board.

Q: Any role models who inspire you?

A: I guess President Barack Obama, who has an amazing ability to remain gracious in the face of extreme hostility. Not only is he capable, but seems to have keen insight into the duties of being President.

At home in a hallway that I pass all the time, I've hung photos taken from the Internet: Barack Obama, Nelson Mandela, Martin Luther King, and Mahatma Gandhi.

Q: How do you arrange the rest of your life to let you do this good work?

A: There's a Zen garden in back of my home with roses, vegetables, a koi pond, and a waterfall. It sits between the open face of a cabana and a wire fence fastened to poles of peeled pine. Over the fence I can see Mount Atalaya. In the cabana are chairs and a couch, side tables and a dining table. When the weather's good, that's where I spend most of my free time, just enjoying being alive. No music, no television. I don't eat breakfast but take my coffee out to the cabana for an hour before heading into work. I don't eat a regular dinner, so grab some food from St. Elizabeth's kitchen, drive home, and if it's warm, sit outside until sundown.

Three or four times a week I visit my second husband, Roger. He's in a nursing home because of primary lateral sclerosis in his right leg, totally useless after a four-year decline. Roger and I have known each other since high school.

Since we're needing to live apart, I've been given more time alone. I go through spurts of keeping a journal and have written poems all my life. I put them in a spiral notebook with a burgundy cover. Sometimes I'll enclose one in a card to my kids or a close friend. Here's a poem I posted on Facebook last August, sweating after weeding the vegetable garden. I didn't want to kill the weeds—they'd just started to flower—but if I wanted veggies, I had to.

Even as I pull the weed
I acknowledge its beauty

I also do a little painting, and hope to do more since recently learning about water-soluble oils—far less clean-up time. Petroglyphs fascinate me, especially the animal-headed ones. I let my imagination go to work. In my living room I've hung a canvas of three antlered, human figures backed by a flaming sky, with cobalt and forest greens in the foreground. Sometimes I use bright colors, sometimes I mute them.

Because I'm pretty good at delegating authority and creating a team environment—trusting employees to make good decisions in my absence—I usually don't need to work on weekends, but I will make presentations. Last weekend I made a twenty-minute appeal for funds at all three services of St. John the Baptist Catholic Church on Osage Avenue. Members of that church serve lunch to the homeless Monday through Friday.

Q: What effect does religious or spiritual practice have on your work?

A: I'm not a religious Buddhist, I'm a meditative Buddhist. I don't go in for chanting the sutras. But I like the methodology of meditation and the concept that we're all one. I was raised German Catholic by my grandparents in the north woods of Minnesota, and have taken to heart Jesus' teachings to feed the hungry and clothe the naked. Since I believe we are one, I believe Jesus and Buddha say the same thing. We must care for those in need.

Once a month, fifteen or twenty other women and I go to a morning retreat at a friend's house for three hours on the Sunday closest to the new moon, which symbolizes our menstrual cycles. We share, we don't read text. In good weather we do a walking meditation.

Q: What disappointments do you deal with in your work?

A: Our budget is $1,400,000 a year, but only thirty percent of that comes from city, state, and federal governments. We've tried to get a greater percentage but it's not working. Federal funding started dropping in 2005, and the loss accelerated in 2012.

Our Sonrisa Family Supportive Living, Casa Cerrillos for adults with disabilities, Siringo Senior Housing, and Casa Familia all appeal to funders. The Men's Emergency Shelter doesn't. The general opinion seems to be that a man should go out and get a job. This mind-set does not take into account mental and physical disabilities.

The biggest challenge is finding money for overhead and administration. Donors to St. Elizabeth's want to support particular programs.

It's a disappointment to see our homeless guests so beaten down by society and turns of events that they've lost hope. Internalized oppression is the term we use for believing that you're unworthy, stupid, and can't make it in this world. Especially this is true for people of color: Native Americans, Hispanics, Blacks; they're most likely to agree with the stereotypes placed on them. We're able to reach out to some, yes, but it's increasingly difficult to serve as many as we'd like to.

Sometimes guests will sabotage themselves, relapse into homelessness after obtaining housing and becoming fairly stable. They stop paying rent, stop going to their jobs, stop taking their meds.

Q: Please share a few examples of your success with the homeless.

A: We have so many of them. Former guests come back to tell us how they're doing.

Probably opening Casa Familia for women and children is my biggest success. Last year we had nine new babies. Some of our mothers were already here, some came from the hospital. As with our men guests, so with the women—we have a respite program, using partial funding from Christus St. Vincent Regional Medical Center. The discharge nurse will call us if a patient leaving has nowhere else to go.

One of our guests had three children. She'd lost her clerking job at a big-box store and, having used up all her savings, been evicted from her apartment. A few months later we helped her find work, and used money from our Good Sam (Samaritan) Fund to share the cost of deposit at another apartment. She and the kids are still there after three years.

Often women and men come to us after surgeries—abdominal, frostbite, heart troubles, amputations. In 2013 the hospital sent us Mark Garcia, not his real name. The surgeon had put pins in his thighs and calves after a car hit him. We called him Bionic Man. The National Guard had discharged Mark honorably, following a tour in Iraq. This qualified him for a pension of fifteen hundred dollars a month. We provided care for six months. By then he was able to leave his wheelchair to walk short distances. We connected him to the Veteran Administration's Supportive Housing program so he could receive vouchers for rent.

Q: How do you go about fund-raising?

A: We stress that we're more than a shelter; we don't just warehouse people. Shelter and food are the first steps, but even though some guests don't want to leave, we help them find self-esteem, permanent housing, and an income stream.

Grantors don't respond to numbers as much as they respond to individual stories. They want to see a positive outcome from the money they're giving. That's why we've produced a six-minute video showcasing family success stories.

Many potential funders think St. Elizabeth's just means the men's shelter. One year, for instance, we asked a city council committee for funds to redo the roof on Siringo Senior Housing. One of the committee's members knew nothing about Siringo or Casa Familia or Casa Cerrillos. Once we filled her in, the council approved funding.

Obtaining funding for St. Elizabeth's five shelters is hard. Unlike a college's alumni or a hospital's former patients, our past guests, however grateful, don't give large donations. A thousand-dollar check is big. Some donors mail in five or ten dollars a month—most people do want to help other people.

Our most successful fund-raiser is the Hungry Mouth Festival, held after hours on a Saturday in October. In 2014 a hundred and sixty people came. Most paid a hundred dollars for an early-bird ticket. The rest had to pay twenty-five dollars more.

Ticket holders sample twelve gourmet dishes—three appetizers, three vegetarian entrées, three meat entrées, and three desserts—prepared from donated ingredients by three celebrity chefs. The chefs from each year become judges the next. Attendees vote, using a ballot. A live band entertains and we hold a silent auction.

In 2014 we raised more than $50,000. The Santa Fe High School basketball team served as set-up crew. The winning vegetarian entrée was green chile enchiladas with rice and beans, and the winning dessert was butterscotch pudding.

Deborah Tang's Thumbnail Bio:

Born in South Haven, Michigan, 1953. BA in Political Science, Oregon State University, 1991. MAs in Community and Regional Planning, and Latin American Studies, University of New Mexico, 1995. Manager, micro-loan portfolio for low-income start-ups in New Mexico, 1995–1997. Executive Director, Navajo United Methodist domestic-violence shelter, 1998–2003. Executive Director, St. Elizabeth Shelter, 2005–present. Co-chair, New Mexico Coalition to End Homelessness, 2001–2009. Co-Chair, New Mexico Behavioral Health, Local Collaborative 1 (Santa Fe, Los Alamos, Rio Arriba counties), 2012–present.

Statistics on Homelessness:

The main cause of homelessness is poverty. Illness can cost a poor person everything. Santa Fe's St. Elizabeth Shelter houses 2,000 of New Mexico's 17,000 homeless. Nationally, an estimated 578,424 people had no place to call home at the beginning of 2014. Of these, 216,197 had families and 362,163 did not. About 15% of them were chronically homeless and 9% were veterans. One out of thirty were children.

According to Amnesty International USA, vacant houses outnumber the homeless five to one.

To Help Out or Get Help:

National

> National Alliance to End Homelessness
> 1518 K Street NW, 2nd Floor
> Washington, DC 20005
> (202) 638-1526
> www.endhomelessness.org

> National Coalition for the Homeless
> 2201 P Street NW
> Washington, DC 20037
> (202) 462-4822
> www.info@nationalhomeless.org

In Santa Fe

New Mexico Coalition to End Homelessness
1219 Luisa Street #2
Santa Fe, NM 87504
(505) 982-9000
www.nmceh.org

St. Elizabeth Shelter
804 Alarid Street
Santa Fe, NM 87505
(505) 982-6611
www.steshelter.org
www.volunteer@steshelter.org

Russel Stolins
FOSTER PARENT

Diane Kell
FOSTER PARENT

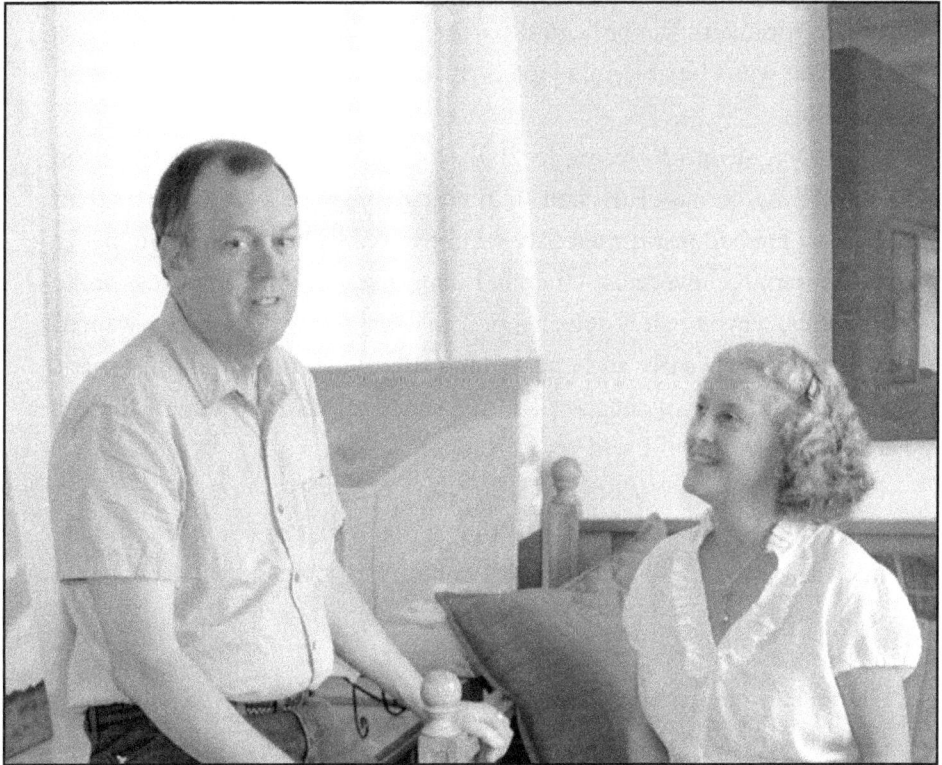

Q: Russel and Diane, tell us what's involved with foster care.

A (Russel): A lot of patience and adaptability, a lot of love, a desire to help kids who have hit bad times. CYFD (New Mexico's Children, Youth, and Families Department) may call at any hour, day or night, asking if we can take a child for twenty-four hours up to a few weeks or even months. We've had kids from five days old to seventeen years old.

A (Diane): I heard at a CYFD meeting that a large percentage of people fostering in New Mexico are grandparents. A second group does it for ethical, religious, or charitable reasons. This group is too small. Then there are those, like Russ and me, who have used foster care as a trial balloon toward adopting. Some of us drop out because we can't find the right match, but we want to keep being helpful. The state's primary goal is reunification with the biological parents. This may take up to two years. If so, you won't be able to adopt even though you've fallen in love with the child.

We got into fostering in 2007, soon after marrying, each for the second time, because Russ had an intense desire to be a father better than his own. He had just turned fifty—I'm five years older—when we met at the Unitarian Universalist Church. In our first year of dating, Russ broke into sobs, maybe half a dozen times, that his first wife had not wanted children. I knew early on he was going to ask me to marry him. I was a widow with a grown daughter and stepson, but realized younger children would be involved if I said yes to Russ.

Russel: Lots of women had had to hear, on a first or second date, how much I wanted to adopt. I couldn't commit to someone who was going to shut that door.

Diane: In order to foster, we completed a home study, long questionnaires about us and our families. A state-appointed therapist interviewed us several times and our backgrounds were checked for criminality. Then we attended several all-day workshops in Española. The instructors talked about differences between non-traumatized kids and foster kids, emphasizing the emotional costs to foster kids of bouncing from home to home. We learned the importance of setting up strict rules, and why corporal punishment is forbidden. One piece of role-playing had us becoming foster kids ourselves. We were asked how it felt to experience relatives and friends gradually disappearing until there was no one left.

Russel: We took kids for weeklong placements until meeting a brother and sister the Christmas week of 2008. The social worker said they were ideal adoptees, that the young girl had manageable asthma and her brother's tantrums were only occasional—but that after two years, their grandmother couldn't cope. The sister was eight and her brother was six, charming, entertaining, bright. Another couple had reneged on promising to become their adoptive parents.

So Diane and I said we'd like to take them on a foster-to-adoption placement. The honeymoon lasted three weeks. The girl began kicking and scratching, punching holes in the walls of her bedroom. She needed multiple trips to the emergency room for breathing and psychiatric problems.

Brother and sister would tag-team their tantrums, one starting as we finally got the other calmed down. CYFD pays for therapy once a week if the children stay more than a month. Their regular therapist, and a specially appointed behavioral therapist, gave us conflicting advice on how best to get the kids settled in our home. But after three months, CYFD determined that the girl needed a higher level of care than we had been trained to provide.

The department moved her into what's called a treatment-foster-care family, agreeing to leave the young boy with us. In just two weeks he became a happy, normal child. Four months later, CYFD decided that brother and sister should be together. We still wanted to adopt both, but we never got to see them again.

Diane: Eight months had elapsed. Russ and I took a break for another four. But we recalled that most of the kids we'd fostered had had no more problems than kids anywhere. I realized I felt like Russ, still hoping to adopt. We told CYFD, however, that for the time being we wanted to be available only for respite care, giving other foster parents time off.

Russel: Like with one boy and his brother, nine and seven. Their biological mom, in a rage, had broken their thumbs. They said they looked forward to staying with us and Nievé, our little dog, while their foster parents took trips. The boys loved throwing a baseball over my head, so I couldn't catch it. Or we'd walk beside the railroad tracks collecting rusty spikes. I teach students at IAIA (the Institute of American Indian Arts) how to create electronic portfolios of their creative writing and artworks, and was able to let the boys play Asteroids on the huge screen of the college's new Digital Dome.

Diane: Russ enjoys kids he can do dad things with: board games, snowball fights, reading a story or poems to them at night, walking Nievé. I like the littlest kids best, cuddling them, rocking and singing them to sleep. They're just so sweet, even when they cry. If they're over three years old, I love doing crafts with them. But trauma disrupts the way their brains are organized. That's what causes the emotional problems. We believe that trying to be caring, thoughtful adults has a positive effect.

Russel: Maybe they'll not remember us as individuals, but we're part of a thread of love that gets them through a harrowing time.

Diane: Here I should say that besides calling us for respite care, CYFD sometimes uses us for forty-eight-hour holds while the police and the agency conduct their initial investigation. For example, two years ago a mentally challenged mom, who herself had grown up in a foster family, left home to be with her boyfriend. He soon got her pregnant. We kept the five-day-old boy for forty-eight hours while CYFD found safe living quarters for both mom and infant. Last year we took a two-year-old for a couple of days because the birth mom was in the hospital. The girl's father had shot her in the neck in a Lowe's parking lot.

Russel: Diane and I do stay open to fostering a child longer than a week. One young girl had come to our home several times, three to five days each, for respite care. We agreed to keep her from January until school let out, thinking we might like her to become a more permanent part of the household.

Diane: In her room she hung a beautiful color photo of herself at eleven, taken for the New Mexico Heart Gallery. This nonprofit posts photos in hospitals, airports, shopping malls, and some art galleries of kids available for adoption. The little girl enjoyed staring at it. "I like to remember myself when young and innocent," she'd say.

One day I found the photo, slashed and the frame broken, stuffed into our trash can. "*You* don't belong in a trash can," I told her. She let me repair it and paint the image so that it became an acrylic portrait. She hung it up again, then started stealing credit-card information. After her graduation from eighth grade, CYFD decided she had a better chance of conquering her demons by living in a group-treatment center. We agreed, although she'd lasted longer with us than with any previous family.

Q: Russel, what life experiences have contributed to your doing this good work?

A: I was raised by a present, mostly loving mother and largely absent father. Though he'd dropped out of John Hopkins University, he found work as an aerospace engineer in Southern California. When I turned four, both parents—for some reason I don't know—became Mormons. Then my father spent even more time away from home, volunteering for the church.

There's an eight-inch-long, yellow race car in my study that I supposedly made as a Cub Scout for Pinewood Derby. It beat out a dozen others, racing down a thirty-foot incline and winning the championship. The car wasn't really mine. It was a way for my father to show his own skill, polishing, for instance, the shafts of nails holding the wheels to reduce friction. The project had nothing to do with showing me how to develop confidence.

He'd often told me that he'd never pay for a college education, that it was a waste of time. So after graduating from high school, I worked at odd jobs, selling cable TV subscriptions, clerking in a bookstore, to accumulate enough money three and a half years later to attend the University of California at Berkeley. By the time I got my BA, I knew I wanted to be a father, remembering so many poor approaches from my parents.

Before I moved north for college, I looked forward to gatherings of four generations on Thanksgiving at my grandmother's home in Santa Monica. Those get-togethers gave me a sense of family. But then my grandparents and great-grandmother moved to the middle of nowhere in Missouri, two hours east of Springfield, to be closer to my grandfather's relatives. I decided the only way to get a sense of family again was to start one of my own.

In my junior year at Cal, helping as a research assistant for the Forest Service, I met this wonderful professor, a wiry Czechoslovakian in his mid-fifties. He conducted management studies. Had I been able to handpick my own father, I'd have chosen him. He didn't give advice, he showed how to ask the right questions, letting me grow at my own pace. As I approached my senior year, he inquired what project I'd like to take on. "Oh, my supervisor will come up with something," I said. "No, man," he said, "what do *you* want to do?"

By age thirty, I still hadn't found a marriage partner, so I embarked on what I thought would be six months of therapy that turned into six years. A major revelation was that I had a much more vivid vision of being a father than of being a spouse.

Q: And Diane, what life experiences have contributed to your doing this good work?

A: It never would have occurred to me to do foster care if I hadn't met Russ. I probably would have thought it foolish, given our ages, except that I had found mothering little kids easy. The teenage years were a different story, one reason I'm sometimes reluctant to take teenagers now.

But Russ was, and is, so good with my grandchildren that I knew he'd be a great foster dad. Even so, after one of our training sessions with CYFD, I got cold feet. Then I imagined three toddlers knocking at our front door and thought, *How can I say no? They need to come in.*

My parents may have been overly strict but very loving. Me becoming a mother was imprinted early on. I played constantly with dolls, personalizing them. When my daughter, Lindsey, from my first husband was young, I wouldn't let her take a doll outside in the winter without dressing the doll warmly.

When Lindsey was seven and in first grade, during an after-school program, she and her best friend were playing jungle gym on a high cart with their stuffed Easter bunnies. A TV set weighing maybe a hundred pounds sat on top. Somehow she tipped the cart over. The TV fell on her head, resulting in a cracked skull and traumatic brain injury. Fire engines, an ambulance, and police cars had all arrived when I, knowing nothing, came to pick her up. The headmaster hurried over to say, "Lindsey's had an accident." It felt as though he'd rammed a phone pole into my chest. "Is she conscious?" I asked. "No," he answered, helping me into a police car to rush to the hospital.

In the emergency room I started shaking uncontrollably. But then I decided, *The doctors can't see me as hysterical. I need to focus on helping Lindsey get well.* She stayed in a coma for two weeks. During that time my only thought was, *All I need is for her to be awake. If she can feel my love, that will be enough. It almost doesn't matter whether she can run or even walk again.* Thank God Lindsey did recover.

Q: Russel, any current role models who inspire you?

A: My fostering really has all been driven by the daily ache of childlessness, though I wouldn't have gotten into fostering without Diane. Her great gift to me is her willingness to help.

At one time, our charges, a fifteen-month-old, and his brother, three months old—arrived with problems. The older boy came with his arm in a cast, and the young needed gastrointestinal surgery. Caring for them was hard work. But done with a loving spouse, it was the shared endeavor I'd always yearned for.

Not only have I discovered Diane's skill and ever-giving heart—for the first time, the ache of childlessness has lessened. I figured I'd have to live with it forever. Before marrying Diane, I drew two timelines, one involving adoption, one not. The line without children took twenty years off my life because of anguish, the sense of failure.

Diane has taught me so many things regarding how to be a father. As patient as my students at IAIA claim me to be, she showed how much more patience effective fostering requires.

Q: And for you, Diane, any current role models?

A: At the time this book was published, Scott, a placement worker at CYFD—tall, with a black ponytail and soothing baritone—is always there for us. Early this year, one boy, a too-thin eight-year-old, who had run to the top of the ridge behind our home, started throwing rocks and breaking limbs. When I tried to get close, he'd back away, screaming. When I sat on the bench without moving, he approached, just like my puppies used to do. I called Scott. He told me to walk back toward the house, that the boy probably would follow. He did, but dashed into the art studio/guest bedroom and began screaming again. Finally he agreed to let Scott calm him down.

One investigative caseworker, who looks like a biker with both arms tattooed, talks to the kids in a matter-of-fact, everything's-under-control manner. Once, when I visited CYFD to pick up a twelve-year-old who'd told the police her father had forced her to fondle him, the caseworker led the girl and me into another room. There, from dozens of bins of clothes, he let her choose outfits for the next two days, explaining I'd be driving her to the University of New Mexico hospital, so a woman doctor could ask questions about sexual abuse.

We aren't well acquainted with other foster parents. Just hearing about those willing to take up to six kids for six to twelve months is inspiring. Last week, I met a foster mom with seven kids, including two babies and two teenagers. I expressed astonishment. She told me she knew someone who had adopted three kids and then took in nine siblings to foster.

Russ's and my usual commitment is one or two children for maybe five days. None of us are making money at this, by the way. We get less than a day-care worker would. For the brothers now with us, we receive five hundred dollars a month for each boy. That hardly covers expenses like diapers, toys, a crib, food. Fostering is not a living, it's a calling.

It pleases and embarrasses me when, buying toys, say, I mention I'm a foster mom, and the clerk exclaims, "Oh, I'm so glad you're doing that!" I don't feel I deserve such praise because others are doing more than Russ and me, and because fostering is a privilege. The babies love you. They gurgle, they laugh. With older kids you give more than you get, but even one "I'm having fun with you" feels good.

Q: Russel, how do you arrange the rest of your life to let you do this good work?

A: There have been two phases. From 2008 to 2011, I worked full time at home writing computer textbooks. Diane worked full time at an art gallery and then for an architect. I did most of the shuttling kids around.

In 2011 I took a full-time position teaching computer and writing skills at IAIA. I'd teach on campus, help with dinner and getting the kids to bed, and teach online afterwards.

In 2013 we had an eighth-grader with us for five months. My routine was to get up at three or four and write until seven. I'd drive her to and from the charter school across from IAIA. It's remarkable how long applying makeup takes while riding in a car!

Q: Diane, what about you? How do you arrange the rest of your life?

A: I put a lot of it on hold. The foster kids usually sleep on a trundle bed in my studio. When we care for children who can reach the top of my art table, I put brushes, canvases, and acrylic paint in the closet.

Often I can paint in spurts, working from the thousands of photos Russ and I have taken of rainbows, sunsets, clear skies, and clouds. At least a dozen sky paintings are hanging in my studio. Caseworkers coming through have commented, "What a nice environment for the children."

When younger kids are here, I put my other passion—gardening— aside or ask Russ to take charge for an hour or two. Last week I was able to plant a climbing iceberg rose, and some red-twig dogwoods under our aspen. When we keep older kids for more than a few days, day care frees times for painting and gardening. My days would quickly fill if I wasn't doing any fostering. Saturdays I used to enjoy running errands with Russ or seeing a movie at The Screen or the Cinemateque. We can't do that anymore. We have taken the two boys to a graduation barbeque for one of Russ's students.

Q: Russel, what effect does religious or spiritual practice have on your foster parenting?

A: It's not as if I've ever felt a religious calling to do this work. I was raised a Mormon and eventually found a home in Unitarianism, though Diane and I became inactive a couple of years after we started to foster. The single most important religious influence on me is Thomas Paine's *The Age of Reason.* He wrote, "My church is the world and my religion is to do good." I take my cues on how to live from that.

For most of my adult life, I've wanted to experience as many facets of being human as I could. I've gone through childhood, I've gone through caring—sometimes for months—for my grandmother in her final years. But until becoming a foster dad, I hadn't witnessed daily the loving nurturing of a child. These foster kids help me see creation through fresh eyes.

Three things seem to make life worth living. One, witnessing the beauty of creation. Two, the loving relationships we can form. And three, art, especially music.

Q: For you, Diane, what effect does religious or spiritual practice have on your fostering?

A: For several years while my daughter was growing up, I taught Sunday school and chaired the religious-education committee at the Unitarian Universalist church. Russ and I met at the UU church here in Santa Fe. Forrest Church, a former Unitarian leader in New York, was well-known for his claim that everyone, whether believing in God or not, has a religion. He said that religion is "our human response to the dual realities of being alive and having to die."

I do often wonder, *What's the point in being alive?* Mostly I think it's about babies—cuddly, their button noses and rosebud cheeks—perfectly designed to be loved. It's a spiritual belief of mine that it's wrong to live only for oneself. More than anything else, fostering makes me feel useful, helping young people to feel cared for. They're growing up with far more difficulties than I had.

Q: Russel, what doubts and disappointments do you deal with in this work?

A: An eleven-year-old I'll call Rosa tested my patience in ways I hadn't experienced. After an hour of trying to persuade her to stop her tantrums, so we all could get some sleep, I walked out of her room and put my fist through a kitchen-cabinet door. Diane later succeeded where I'd failed. I told myself, *I just don't have what it takes.*

Then there was one boy, a thirteen-year-old with a blond mop of hair. Diane had grown afraid of him because he'd thrown a couple of books at her. We urged the caseworker to place him with another family, but CYFD had already decided he should learn social skills at a residential treatment enter. I argued that he only needed a lot of family love. His bio father had murdered his bio mother, he'd lived for two days with the corpse, his adopted mother had beat and then abandoned him. Afterward he'd bounced from home to home.

The center he ended up in, near El Paso, was miles from anyone who cared about him. He phoned us every day for six months. We made three seven-hundred-mile trips to see him in the center's cafeteria; we weren't allowed private visits.

CYFD later placed him in a treatment foster home fifty miles east of us, but we were never allowed to see or talk with him again. So frustrating!

Q: Diane, what doubts and disappointments do you deal with?

A: Most of our kids are sweet and fun and good. But we've cared for a few with severe behavioral problems. I worry, *Am I putting myself in a situation that could be dangerous?*

One girl, for example, was only eleven and small, but violent. We had to put the kitchen knives up high. Russ and I read everything we could find on Reactive Attachment Disorder. One of the features is that the child misbehaves only at home; she was a model student. The emotional stress on all three of us was awful for six weeks before CYFD moved her out.

The caseworker told us not to share, on the last morning, that we weren't driving her to school but to the therapist's home for transfer. She soon figured this out. She had a major meltdown in the back, biting her wrists and screaming. I told Russ to keep driving and climbed over the seat. When I tried to hold her in my arms, she bit into my forearm. When we arrived, I was afraid she'd run away if I opened the door, so I waited in the car with her. Minutes later, the therapist and caseworker rushed out to help.

Q: Russel, how about examples of successes?

A: There have been some really good moments. Here I am, at this time, sixty years old, and last month, for the first time, I got to show off a baby. I kept him on campus for a couple of hours. In the cafeteria, maybe a dozen IAIA students and half a dozen faculty fawned over him, expressing so much gratitude that I'm caring for him. Many didn't know that side of me, that I'm a foster dad.

One of our toughest placements was a girl who didn't believe anyone loved her, wouldn't let anyone close. We kept her for six months, though we couldn't help her find the self-discipline she required to get along in the world. We did recommend Albuquerque's residential treatment center and that seemed to work. She became open to being adopted by her Rio Rancho foster family.

A few years back we gave three Navajo siblings a stable home for three weeks: a girl, twelve, a boy, nine, and another boy, five. Their mom was in the Esperanza Shelter for Battered Families. Every day Diane or I would drive the kids in from Eldorado and across town to Agua Fria Elementary. The two older ones were pretty obese. We made sure they all ate healthy foods and got complete physicals and eye exams at the Indian Hospital. To improve their stamina, we took them on hikes. Meanwhile, CYFD searched for a family member through tribal authorities. An uncle at Fort Defiance, in Arizona's Navajo Nation, finally took the children.

We've all heard of unrequited love; there's also unrecorded love. That's what Diane and I are giving these kids. They may not remember us. Their bio parents don't know us. Mostly the only record of our love for them is between Diane and myself. Yet we're part of their lives now, part of reversing the cycle of grown-ups letting them down.

Q: Diane, a couple more successes?

A: We took a fourteen-year-old Native American who'd been raised in foster homes since the age of four. Toward the end of her stay, she told the

caseworker, "Diane understands me without my having to say anything."
I said, "If you want to live the life you've talked about—going to college,
raising a happy family, being respected—you need to deal with whatever
leads you to steal credit cards in order to visit adults-only chat rooms for
sexually suggestive conversations with strange men." I suspect I was the
first person to see that her problems had their root in early childhood
sexual trauma.

I suggested sending her to a residential treatment center where she
could share her past with a professional. She laid her head on the table
and wailed, "I'll do it, I want to go!" When Russ and I visited her in
Albuquerque one time, she said the therapist was the only one she'd ever
felt safe in opening up to.

So far, caring for the two boys feels like a success. I take them to the
CYFD office in Santa Fe three days a week for an hour's visit with their
biological mom and dad, who attend parenting classes and are meeting
other requirements to get their sons back. The boys don't cry in the car,
going to see their parents or coming home. They seem to feel safe and
happy with us, but are still attached to their parents. After each visit, a
client-services associate comes out with the parents to the parking lot. I
tell their mom and dad what games Russ and I and the boys have been
playing, or news about the latest doctor's appointment.

Russel Stolins's Thumbnail Bio

Born in Los Angeles, California, 1955. BA Anthropology, UC Berkeley, 1980. Speakers-bureau volunteer coordinator, suicide prevention hotline, 1981–1984. MA Educational Technology, San Francisco State University, 1991. Wrote first textbook, *Laying a Foundation with Windows 95,* 1996. Full-time textbook author, 1999-2011, twenty-plus titles published. Taught writing and/or computer skills at Vista Community College, Berkeley, 1984–1997; UC Berkeley Extension, 1992–1998; San Francisco State University, 1995–1997; Santa Fe Community College, 1999–2012; Institute of American Indian Arts, 2012–present. Home study to become adoptive parent with first wife, 2001. Received adoption/foster-parent license, 2008. Estimated children fostered to date, 60, ranging in age from 5 days old to 17 years.

Diane Kell's Thumbnail Bio

Born in East Lansing, Michigan, 1950. BA Art History, Brown University, 1972. EdM, Harvard Graduate School of Education, 1996; began EdD, degree not completed. Chair, Religious Education Committee, Unitarian Universalist Church, Lexington, Massachusetts, 1984–1987. Board Member and Chair, Education Committee, Fayerweather Street School, Cambridge, Massachusetts, 1984–1988. LewAllen Galleries' administrator and marketing coordinator, 2005–2009. Began fostering, 2008. Atkin Olshin Schade Architects, administrator and marketing coordinator, 2010–2012. Painted watercolors, 1997–2002. Painted skies in acrylics, 2013–present.

Statistics on Foster and Adoptive Children to Date:

Of the 450,000 children in foster care nationally, 21% will be adopted and 51% will be reunified with their parents or primary care givers, according to the National Foster Care Coalition. Their median age is 8.5 years and 52% are male. 47% live with non-relatives and 28% with relatives. At present, 110,000 foster children are waiting to be adopted.

In New Mexico, 1,900 children are in foster care, with 133 heading toward adoption. 60% will be reunified with their natural families within twelve months; only 12% are expected to reenter foster care.

To Learn How to Become a Foster or Adoptive Parent:

National

    National Foster Care Coalition
    www.nationalfostercare.org

    National Foster Parent Association
    www.nfpaonline.org

    Adopt Us Kids
    www.adoptuskids.org

In Santa Fe

    Children, Youth, and Families Department
    For general information, log onto www.cyfd.org
    To foster or adopt a child, call (800) 432-2075

Tony McCarty
Executive Director, Kitchen Angels

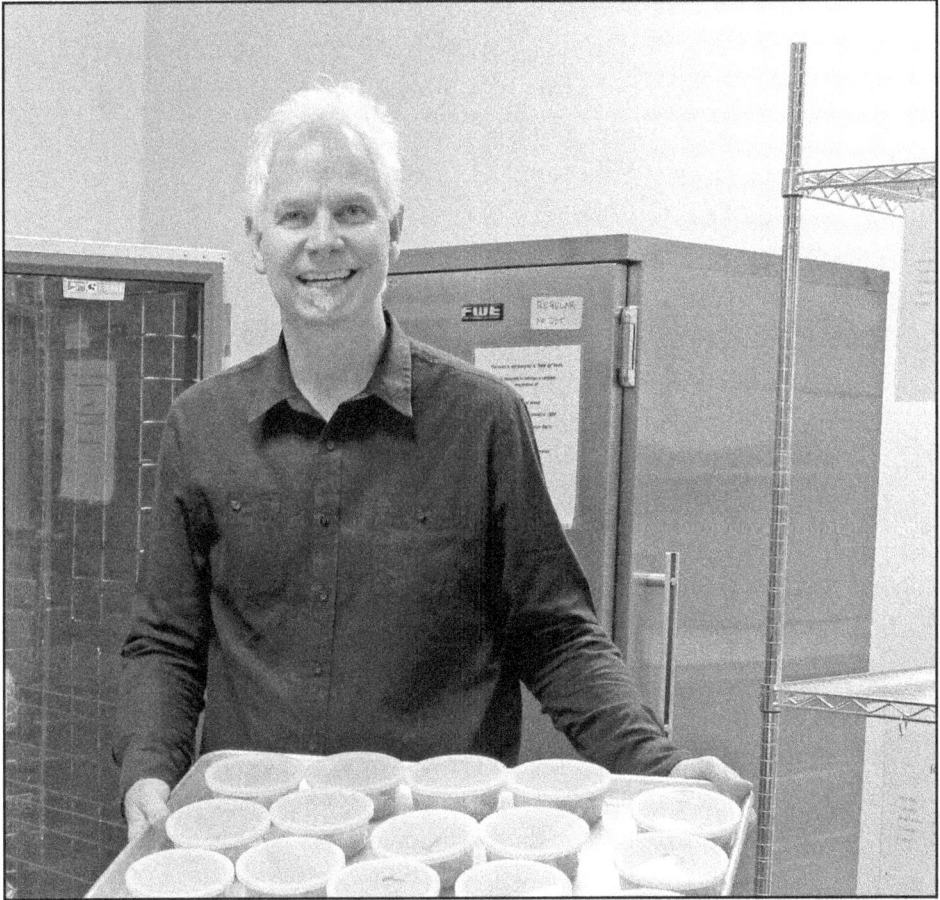

Q: Tony, what is Kitchen Angels all about?

A: We're a nonprofit founded in 1992, cooking—and delivering in the evenings—free hot meals on weekdays, and frozen meals for weekends to four hundred homebound clients ineligible for other food programs.

Ninety-eight percent of these folks live below the Federal Poverty Guidelines and half, our fastest growing percentage, are seniors on special diets. Without Kitchen Angels, most of them would face homelessness or life in a nursing home paid for by someone else.

I'll tell you a story that changed my perception of the program. When I'd been here five years, and was the only employee, one of our volunteer drivers called in sick. So I took over. At my third delivery, the door opened partway and a thin hand reached out for the meal. I decided to ask, "How are you feeling today?"

"You mean you'd like to visit?" a voice asked.

I said, "Yes."

"Come on in," he said, and turned on a gigantic fountain in the middle of the room, surrounded by a bunch of potted plants. He was in his early twenties and, it turned out, one of New Mexico's first identified cases of AIDS. His family had abandoned him. That's the day I learned that our mission is not all about food. Human contact is just as important.

Q: What are your duties now?

A: Everything—or find others to help. I'm on call twelve, fourteen hours a day, to keep the funding going and make sure I do the will of the Board. Volunteer Board members come to headquarters once a month, expecting to stay at least a couple of hours. Each of these good people also heads up a committee, Strategic Planning, Finance, Fund-raising/Events, seven more.

My day often starts with appointments. As one of the founders of Santa Fe's Food Policy Council, I'll meet members for breakfast. Our Board's Marketing Committee also likes breakfasting out. I'm especially keen on being a guest on early-morning radio to reach the rush-hour crowd.

In the office, I'll first check with our few paid staff. Right now Teresa Norton heads up our kitchen, Jeanette Iskat makes sure our homebound clients are getting their dietary needs met, and Lauren LaVail oversees our volunteer cooks and drivers and serves as community liaison.

Next I'll deal with emails and consult with some of our three hundred and forty-five volunteers. Passionate interaction is why Kitchen Angels has held my imagination all these years. Last week one of our drivers found her client unconscious on the front steps. She called 911, and waited for the ambulance. The next day she delivered Gatorade and a hot lunch—and stayed to talk.

My favorite volunteers are teenagers that the Teen or Municipal Court, because of misbehavior at school, has assigned mandatory community service. I know that by the end of the day, the kids most pissed off at having to spend time here are going to be smiling. Why? Because of being surrounded by volunteers who love what they're doing. There's an immediate reward in cooking and delivering food. When Teresa, our kitchen manager, tells a kid, "Pull up your pants and next time wear a belt," he does it, no questions asked. We've even had some who return on their school vacations to help out.

A couple of mornings a week the bookkeeper appears. I have to make sure the bills are paid and that the monthly financial reports to the Board are accurate. And there's always planning and grant-writing to be done. I also write most of our newsletter.

Mornings and afternoons are peppered with interruptions. The guy designing a logo for our reconditioned-cookware store, the musician wanting his band to do a fund-raiser for us, the potential donor, all expect their questions to be answered right now. Sadly that's not always possible. Often I just lunch at my desk. Today I've fixed carrot and sweet potato soup, flavored with ginger and coconut oil. I want to try it out for our kitchen.

Because of our Capital Campaign, I've been lunching with people whose names I've only known from their checks. Or I'll call my laughing partner on the Marketing Committee, Carmon McCumbee, to join me. Her attitude is always, "I'm here to help. What do you need doing?" We talk a little business but mostly we laugh, unbeatable for relaxing. After lunch I return phone calls. That usually takes up an hour and a half, unless

I can shuttle some to staff. I may *think* about a nap but that's it. The rest of the day is taken up with writing chores or looking over reports. On Wednesdays Tim Bock arrives to solve computer problems with our software, website, or Internet phone system, and consult about equipment we need to budget for. He stays at least three hours.

Past five p.m. there are fund-raisers, cocktails at donors' homes, and awards ceremonies. One week Christus St. Vincent Regional Medical Center awarded us some money because our healthy meals keep clients out of the emergency room. You always want to make time to pick up a check like that but not devour so many hors d'oeuvres that you can't eat a decent meal.

I guess I'm a little insane because still, after twenty-two years, every time I arrive at one of our events, I love being there, knowing how many of our homebound clients depend on us for survival.

When I get home, I walk the best dog ever, a cairn-terrier mix from the shelter, have dinner, wind down, and read myself to sleep. I'm about to pick up *Powers of Two* that I heard about on NPR (National Public Radio), how the success of inventions is usually due to two people. That's how things work at Kitchen Angels. Someone comes up with the idea and someone else runs with it.

Q: What life experiences have contributed to your doing this good work?

A: My dad, an industrial machinist in Augusta, Georgia, and very active in the Church of God, had three gardens going—at our house, at my grandmother's, and at my aunt's. Dad just took care of people. He harvested corn, field peas, tomatoes, cucumbers, green beans, watermelons, squash, and gave the excess to the widow on the corner or others in need. I confess that his being so busy annoyed me as a child, but the bigness of his heart made a lasting impression.

Mom worked at least forty hours a week as a seamstress. But she was even more a caregiver than my dad. She and five sisters living nearby scheduled twenty-four-hour care to any other family members or friends who were ill or dying. My grandmother and grandfather died at home, thanks to my mother.

But I was desperate to leave Georgia's hot, hundred-percent-humidity summers. A friend invited me to visit Seattle in August, 1979. Those two weeks of clear skies and temperatures in the mid-seventies made up my mind. I gave notice to the principal at the junior high where I'd been teaching art history for three years since college. Mom said, "You couldn't move any further away and still stay in the United States."

In Seattle I befriended a woman named Barbara Osborne, a writer and artist who offered to rep my jewelry. We cooked for each other every other Wednesday night, then we started cooking for friends. We started to discuss intent: what effect did we want our meals to have? Healing? Seduction? Parental love? Festivity? All I'd learned from my mother and dad, and talks with Barbara, set me up for joining Kitchen Angels.

My two best male friends in Seattle had always wanted to live in Santa Fe, and after one was diagnosed with full-blown AIDS, they moved there. So I began to visit, and thought they'd gone out of their minds. Seattle had everything: cool temperatures, great gardening.

On my last visit, though, walking up Canyon Road, I suddenly got why they'd relocated. The adobe buildings, the light filtering through the giant cottonwoods, the four hundred years of Spanish influence, even the disintegrating sidewalks—there's no place like it.

When one of the two went into the hospital late October of 1992, his partner called, asking for help. I arranged to stay with him for three months. He died two weeks later. I'd been taking a course on how to aid the dying, and at graduation, five nonprofits made presentations, looking for volunteers. I signed up to cook Tuesday afternoons for the newly formed Kitchen Angels.

Cooking on Thursdays and Fridays followed. I realized my life in Santa Fe was becoming more anchored than my life in Seattle. So I sold my house there.

After helping with a successful fund-raiser we called A Picnic in the Style of Monet, I was asked to join the Board. My first paying job, Kitchen Manager, led to becoming Executive Director in 1994.

Q: Any current role models who inspire you?

A: Sarah Taylor, named a Santa Fe Living Treasure in 2013. Her birthday's a day after mine. Before moving here, she ran a cookware store in Bakersfield, The Panhandler. She wears her hair in a salt-and-pepper pageboy, is maybe five-foot-two with a sparkling laugh. A real confidante and gourmet cook who has never cooked for our clients, though she's volunteered in our office for sixteen years and was a Board member for nine. She's one of those people who looks around to see what needs doing, or anticipates what needs to be done, and makes sure it happens. Always there to step forward as a leader.

Q: How do you arrange the rest of your life to let you do this good work?

A: I'm very good at compartmentalizing. It lets me focus on the task at hand. Some people love that ability in me, some hate it. But there's never a complete separation between work and fun for me because I've met my best friends through Kitchen Angels.

My most enjoyable off-work activity is the Sunday Supper Club. Seven of us choose a cuisine, set a menu, get together in rotating homes once a month, and cook.

One Saturday we fixed a sixty-first birthday dinner for me. It took three hours to prepare the dishes and another five to enjoy them. Anchovy fillets with guindilla peppers and garlic-stuffed olives, washed down with lemon-syrup-and-gin-spiked champagne, started us off. Zinfandel of beef, braised pearl onions, sautéed mushrooms, and claret followed, plus a salad of radicchio, arugula, and apple slices. Sound good? We ended with hazelnut meringues layered with bittersweet-chocolate ganache and mocha-butter cream.

Bob Horwitz and I have been together for years. He retired as Chief

Financial Officer for New Mexico's Department of Public Health. On the first day the state legalized same-sex weddings, August twenty-third of 2013, Bob phoned me at work. "Want to get married?" he asked.

"I'm not dressed for the press," I answered flippantly. We met at the courthouse that afternoon.

Bob and I are keen on home-improvement projects and we like to travel, too, especially walking tours.

Q: What effect does religious or spiritual practice have on your work?

A: Our official history describes Kitchen Angels as being "conceived in a flash of divine synchronicity." Before moving here, one of our founders, Tony D'Agostino, volunteered for Project Angel Food in LA, itself founded by the woman who conceived A Course in Miracles. Tony and two others advertised in *The New Mexican* that they needed help starting a hot-meal service for shut-ins in Santa Fe. Thirty people showed up and in less than a month they were cooking and delivering food.

Soon after accepting the job of Executive Director, I felt overwhelmed. So I called Tony D. "What do I do?" I asked him. "Ask the angels," he said. Ever since I've come to trust that they'll send the answer in the form of a person or event. Here's a story:

One of our purveyors brought us a huge side of beef after we'd ordered just a cut of brisket. It couldn't be returned. I totally freaked out. "Give me a little time," our chef said. In an hour and a half she walked into my office holding a tenderloin. "Follow me." In the kitchen she pointed out brisket she'd butchered for the day's meals, stew meat for tomorrow's meals, and tenderloins for a special event.

The big lesson I've learned is to let go of control and let someone else take over. The miracle is, it gets done. Everything goes back to having faith. I try to do this work with an open heart, clearing out all the junk while driving to headquarters.

Q: What doubts and disappointments do you deal with?

A: Kitchen Angels works because everybody does what's assigned—ego has to take a back seat. Newcomers get the easiest tasks. We had a well-known caterer wanting to help. Some pears needed cooking, to ease clients' digestion. Instead of complaining that the task was beneath him, he poached the pears till they turned a beautiful rose-violet, and stuck a mint leaf onto each. This is the attitude we're looking for.

When a regular driver has to cancel, we ask one of our driver co-ordinators—who normally pack the right meal for every client into the vehicles—to take over. They know this is part of their commitment.

Doubts mostly involve funding. One year we had three disasters in a row—the Philippine tsunami, Hurricane Sandy, flooding in Haiti— each just before a funding appeal or event. Money to disaster areas flowed but contributions to Kitchen Angels fell off. Election years drain funding, too.

Q: Other examples of your successes?

A: In 2008, six of us founded the Santa Fe Food Policy Council, devoted to asking officials to pass ordinances that create a sustainable food system for our community. One day we presented our Food Plan to some of them, to Mayor Javier Gonzales, and to the press. Mayor Gonzales expressed special interest in expanding urban agriculture, healthy school lunches, and public transportation direct to grocery stores. The following Tuesday, county commissioners voted unanimously to adopt the Plan. Very few counties around the country have a plan like this in place. Our twenty-five page, full-color booklet gives details.

There's a man in town who for decades has owned a community farm, a big chunk of land that reaches from the river to the Alameda. When we celebrated John's hundredth birthday, he arrived in a golf cart and, under a huge cottonwood, transferred to a wheelchair. Shock of white hair, full white beard.

At the start of every year he'd call asking, "What would you like us to grow for Kitchen Angels?" But a few years ago a friend came into my office to say John had been confined to bed. Could we help out with some meals? "Of course we can help," I said. After a month of consistent nutrition, he was up and supervising activities on his farm again.

Q: How do you go about fund-raising?

A: For the past four years, Kitchen Angels, the Farmers Market Institute, and Home Grown New Mexico have sponsored cooking classes, Local Organic Meals on a Budget. We move the shelving and tables from the kitchen—it's a lot of work—and invite a celebrity chef to facilitate. Participants pay twenty-two dollars for a two-hour session, 5:30 to 7:30. That includes dining on what we cook. Social media and our email list bring people in.

We also present an annual No-Show Ball. The 2014 invitation read, "All dressed up and no place to go—finally! A fancy ball that you don't have to attend." On the inside, a three-stanza poem ends, "Sit back and relax,/ You've done a good deed./ You've sent Kitchen Angels your check./ You've fed those in need!" We enclosed a self-addressed envelope and simple form to fill out. It's a win-win deal because you're probably sick of galas, and we don't incur the expense.

In 2014, as each year, Kitchen Angels hosted four Adventures à la Carte, costing guests seventy-five to a hundred-fifty dollars each. The Valles Caldera National Preserve tour let forty guests explore, by SUV and foot, the world's most perfect inactive volcanic crater, plus enjoy a gourmet picnic. Tea in the Author's Garden found thirty guests strolling Sallie Bingham's five gardens before relaxing with afternoon tea and delicacies while she read from her latest book.

Exploring the Night Skies involved a gourmet dinner at a donor's hacienda, then peering through a telescope under the home's retractable roof. Cavedigger was our most unusual adventure. First we had breakfast at Kitchen Angels, then we drove forty-five miles north to Embudo on the Rio Grande to explore one of the cathedral-like caves that sculptor Ra Paulette has been digging into sandstone cliffs for twenty-five years. We paused for lunch prepared with local produce.

We've staged golf tournaments, and held road-rally treasure hunts, but our signature fund-raiser is Angels Night Out every April. On a designated Thursday at least thirty restaurants give a quarter of their evening take to us. Diners get a fabulous meal in a party atmosphere; we get funding, new volunteers, and new donors; and the restaurants receive good PR, additional patrons, and two turnovers a night. It's a huge undertaking. Sixty volunteers pair up to become ambassadors, two to each eatery. They welcome diners and tell them about Kitchen Angels.

Tony McCarty's Thumbnail Bio:

Born in Augusta, Georgia, 1953. BA in Art Education, Augusta College, 1976. Flat-glass fabricator and fused-glass jewelry designer, 1980–1985. Owner/contractor of Toney Residential Design, 1984–1992. Executive Director, Kitchen Angels, Inc., 1994–present. Cofounder/Vice Chair: Santa Fe Food Policy Council. Founding Committee: Local Organic Meals on a Budget. Advisory Board: Greenhouse Grocers Co-op.

Statistics pertinent to Kitchen Angels:

A growing, elderly population means more people need more health care, assisted living, and social services. Feeding the homebound helps keep them out of emergency rooms and nursing homes, or off the streets.

Enrollment in Kitchen Angels' services has been growing at 18% a year—400 clients in 2014. Ninety-eight percent live below Federal Poverty Guidelines. Forty percent of these have special dietary needs. Cancer, brain disorder, and diabetes are the greatest reasons for their disabilities. Compared to the $75,000 a nursing home costs each year, it costs Kitchen Angels only $1,775 to feed a client who's homebound.

To Help Out, or Get Help:

To give service in the kitchen or as a driver, to alert staff to a homebound potential client in Santa Fe, or to learn how to start a Kitchen-Angels-like facility in your own city, make contact as follows:

Kitchen Angels
1222 Siler Road
Santa Fe, NM 87507

(505) 471-7780
www.kitchenangels.org
info@kitchenangels.org

To learn about the Santa Fe Food Policy Council's Food Plan for increasing access to healthy food over three years, log onto www.SantaFeFoodPolicy.org

Jane Clarke, PhD
Infant Mental Health Specialist

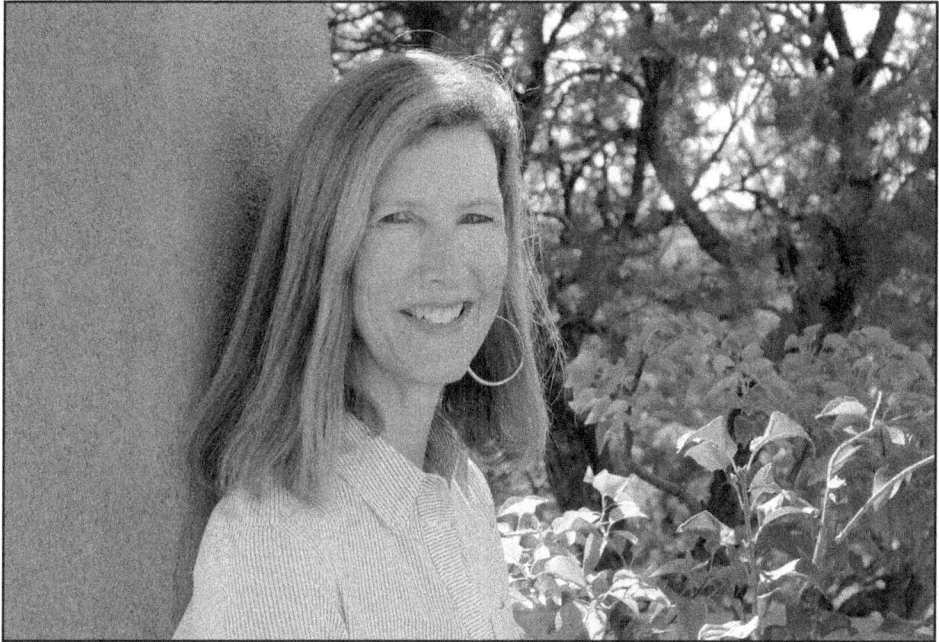

Q: How do you spend your work week, Jane?

A: In four ways. Right now, first of all, Deborah Harris, she's an independent, licensed social worker, and I lead the Infant Team of New Mexico's First Judicial District: Santa Fe, Rio Arriba, and Los Alamos counties. We also consult Infant Teams in Albuquerque, Silver City, and Las Cruces. These teams of specialists provide services for infants and toddlers whom the state has taken in because of maltreatment or neglect.

Our very first case, in 2008, involved a baby exposed to alcohol and drug abuse in the womb. The mother was schizophrenic and the father, with a history of using four or five aliases, was a thief. They fought much of the time. As high as one hundred percent of small children exposed to parental quarrels develop PTSD (post-traumatic stress disorder).

The state's Children, Youth, and Families Department (CYFD) took the infant into custody after a twenty-four-hour investigation, placed him with foster parents, and called Deborah and me. Our assessment always follows two paths. First we look for skin-color changes, breathing patterns, digestive abnormalities, and sensitivities to temperature. This tells us how well the child adapts to changing environments and sensory stimuli. Our little boy was constipated, waked easily, and spit up a lot after finishing his bottles.

Secondly, we look at muscle tone, coordination, and how stiff or relaxed the arm and leg movements are. Our little boy became easily distressed; his muscles quickly stiffened.

Another aspect of our assessment is to have the biological parents come into the CYFD office several times to learn their baby's developmental needs, and so we can observe their social interactions. We also have the foster parents come in, by themselves. Our little boy's biological dad did not appear. He was wanted in Arizona, California, and New Mexico for larceny, stealing cars, and driving under the influence.

The goal of all this is to reunite mother and baby, though often it's not possible. Our little boy's mother could not meet CYFD's mandate to find stable housing—she was homeless—or find a job, or agree to practice making her baby feel safe. So he stayed with his foster parents until the First District's judge decided they could adopt him. I'm still in touch. He's six now and doing very well.

I also consult for New Vistas (pronounced Veestas) Early Intervention Services, a nonprofit agency in Santa Fe. To be eligible, a baby must be twenty-five percent behind normalcy in thinking and motor skills, communication, social skills, and emotional self-regulation. Here I team with Jeanne Du Rivage, an occupational therapist, to do evaluations and make recommendations.

The success of early relationships sets the stage for all future ones. New Vistas called me in to observe a fourteen-month-old girl who kept withholding her breath and turning blue. The mother, it turned out, was afraid to cradle her.

At a toy store now defunct I found a large, round-bottomed, plastic bowl. I coached the mother how to place her baby in it, giving both a needed sense of autonomy. She learned how to rock the bowl with the baby in it, side to side, forward and back, while singing "Twinkle, Twinkle," and "Row, Row, Row Your Boat." Because the mother learned to enjoy herself, so did her infant. They developed more eye contact and expressions of joy.

The father was even more anxious about his baby's welfare than the mom. He had another child in South America and no money to visit.

In addition to our time on the Infant Team, Deb Harris and I teach social workers, child-development therapists, mental-health administrators, and psychiatrists how best to work with traumatized infants and toddlers—eight daylong seminars in the Center for Development and Disability at UNM (University of New Mexico).

Deb and I feel so passionate to spread the word that loving relationships between child and caregiver are key to their mental health that we'll accept invitations from anywhere to speak. So far we've led half-day seminars in Florida, New Hampshire, and Northern California. The oldest participant in our California group was Deb's mother, Ellen, a petite, white-haired social worker who helps the poor cope in San Francisco's Mission District. She was there to gather continuing-education credits in order to renew her license. She's ninety-one and her husband, Ellis, is hell-bent to reach a hundred—he's ninety-nine.

Finally, I make time for one private client, Andy, now eleven, who's in love with high-performance Bugatti cars. At age two-and-a-half, Andy was misdiagnosed with autism. By then he'd suffered through four back surgeries. I was infuriated by the autism label. What he had was medical trauma. Curvature of the spine still causes him physical limitations.

Andy's parents, living in Santa Fe, called me when he'd reached three, no longer eligible for the state's early-intervention services. The family decided to relocate to the Bay Area, to attend Barbara Kalmanson's special-needs school in Marin County. It concentrates on working with traumatized young children. Within a week the parents had put their house up for sale. Though Andy's mother fell into depression, Andy flourished. The family felt able to return to Santa Fe, where the mother's depression disappeared.

Andy's tall for eleven, cheerful, curious about life, a jokester. Once a week we walk the arroyo, play tennis, or go swimming. I've set aside a room in my home where Andy learns social skills. He uses toy cars and wooden people to play out ordinary experiences, like going to see a car mechanic or entering a hospital. He becomes Bob and I'm Jim.

Q: What life experiences have contributed to your doing this good work?

A: My father fell off a stone wall when I was three, and died soon after of a massive cerebral hemorrhage. I was in the living room when a neighbor brought Mother the news. Much later I learned that Dad had been drinking.

He'd doted on me. Ever since then I wanted to disappear, not be seen when conflict arose. That early trauma impacted my relationships until I got a year and a half of therapy in my forties. Always one foot in a relationship and one foot out, because of my fear of abandonment.

Throughout my growing up, Mother devoted herself to others. She recruited four other women in my hometown of Suffield, Connecticut, to help her transport the poor to medical and dental appointments. She found food and clothing for a couple of dozen needy families. People would call her for advice even though she had no credentials except a sympathetic heart. She was forty when she had me, and died fifty years later. This is making me so sad, remembering.

When I was five, I came downstairs to find four hobos at our kitchen table. Mother was serving eggs and bacon and toast while lecturing them to take better care of their families, to be more in touch with their mothers, to give up drinking. She was brought up well-to-do but never turned her back on anyone. Thanks to her I find it easy to get along with people on all socioeconomic levels.

During my years in high school, MacDuffie's School for Girls in Springfield, Massachusetts, I taught inner-city kids—five of them—how to read. Particularly I remember an African-American nine-year-old whose father was in prison for burglary. Every other week for two years I went to his home. We all became close, his mother, his brother, him, and two sisters. I was taken by their struggles; they hoped he'd go to college. I felt I was making a positive difference sometimes just by listening.

Then there's Alicia Lieberman's book, *Losing a Parent to Death in the Early Years*, that I read twenty years ago. It's what persuaded me to get into therapy. Tell the child why the parent's gone. Be honest. Say it's not the child's fault that the parent died or left. Be sure to say, "Your dad, your mom, loved you."

Alicia comes from Paraguay. She's now Vice Chair of the Psychiatry Department at the University of California in San Francisco. At the city's general hospital, she directs the Child Trauma Research Program and the Early Trauma Treatment Network. Deb and I consult with her by phone twice a month.

Q: Any other role models who inspire you?

A: Dr. T. Berry Brazelton, considered the country's premier pediatrician focusing on infants, is in his mid-nineties. I first met him in 1990 while studying for my PhD. He's tall, blue-eyed, bent over a bit, has a toothy smile, loves to dress colorfully—blue pullover sweaters, pink shirts. He taught at Harvard and established the Child Development Unit at Children's Hospital in Boston. I got to know him better in my post-doc studies at the University of Massachusetts. Any baby would want to be held by this guy. They climb all over him. And he makes parents feel successful. It's his smile, I think, and his loving nature, free of judgment.

I used to call him at 8:30 every morning to ask about an infant and family I was working with. The parents had adopted a little girl from

Guatemala who woke up every hour at night to drink a bottle of milk. The father was afraid to just let her cry, because his own mother and dad had left him alone night after night. When the parents are afraid, the baby grows afraid. Dr. Brazelton reminded me to reassure the father that he was a great dad, very caring. And told me ways both parents could reassure their baby, mainly by talking to and holding her.

Dr. Julie Larrieu, a child psychiatrist at Tulane University in New Orleans, helps Deb and me run the Infant Team, decide which parents can probably get their babies back, select evidence to present to the court. A few years ago, in 2012, the state took a nine-month-old boy into custody because his mother was a heroin addict and alcoholic. Domestic violence also caused problems. We asked Julie if she thought the father and mother—she'd been clean and sober for two years—could handle the return of her toddler. The child isn't as coordinated as normal children and has a cleft palate. He says "duh" and points, rather than using words. Can the parents, after counseling, refrain from behavior that will trigger a repeat of making him feel unsafe? It's crucial to have a mentor like Julie, who has so much experience, help us think through difficult cases.

Q: How do you arrange the rest of your life to let you do this good work?

A: It's very important to find a balance, spend enough time with my husband, my daughters, my good friends. And I need exercise. Movement helps me manage stress. Hiking, camping—nature has a calming effect. Twice a week I play tennis with friends or with Challen, my daughter. When I'm in San Francisco, I play in Buena Vista Park with my younger daughter, Hadley.

Listening to folk music and rock—the Fleet Foxes, Radiohead, Smashing Pumpkins—picks me up. A special treat was hearing Wynton Marsalis playing trumpet once at the Lensic.

Probably I spend three hours a day on the computer or reading. Much of that time goes into researching more effective ways to help infants in my care and their families find healthier ways to live. I read for pleasure, too. I've just finished the five fantasy novels in George R.R. Martin's *A Song of Fire and Ice*.

Even though usually I rise at 5:30, I try to get eight hours of sleep. If I can squeeze in a twenty-minute afternoon nap, that's great.

Q: What effect does religious or spiritual practice have on your work?

A: My practice as a Buddhist lets me demonstrate compassion, and keeps me open to the truth that people can change. Plus that we're all connected. It allows me to see the families I work with as no different than myself, with similar drives and needs, especially the need for love.

Once when I was back east, walking after dinner with my cousins under the reds and yellows of huge maples, my cell phone rang. It was one of my mothers, calling to say she'd just been released after a month in Santa Fe's detention center. It hadn't been the first time she'd lost her toddler and her five-year-old to the state because of domestic violence and substance abuse.

She said that she wanted to work with me to get her kids back from foster parents. Instead of being annoyed that she'd called on a Saturday evening, or jaded that she'd gotten clean and sober many times before, I asked my cousins to walk ahead, and stood beside a department store window for half an hour, sharing her dream and coming up with the steps needed to make that dream real.

I've been a Buddhist since 1998. Mostly what I practice is becoming mindful that I don't harm myself or others through wrongful actions or speech. My husband, Clint, and I attend the Upaya Zen Center, ten acres overlooking the Santa Fe River. Roshi Joan Halifax, the abbot and our dear friend, has taught us how to integrate social action with meditation.

Five times a week for half an hour I engage in walking meditation in our foothills and arroyos. Clint and I attend dharma talks together, teachings of the Buddha, such as how fear separates us and makes us more self-absorbed. Also ways to minimize suffering, especially that caused by discontent. All this helps me sort out what I can change and what I can't.

Q: What doubts and disappointments do you deal with in your work?

A: Deb Harris and I look for what we call "good-enough" parenting for babies that CYFD has taken into custody. Sometimes we feel the judge allows the blood parents to take their children back too soon.

A few weeks ago we worked with a mother who had suffered sexual abuse, been a foster-care child, then lived at Girls Ranch, a home for juvenile delinquents. She had lost her two-year-old and one-year-old to the state. Though she was a kind person, and everyone liked her, we found that she couldn't imagine what her children were feeling, even anticipate their basic needs—preparing meals or getting them to sleep at a consistent time. But the judge allowed her to bring them home.

The mother's foster-care sister, a fervent churchgoer, tried to help out by cleaning house, buying groceries, babysitting while the mother looked for work. But the kids stayed unbathed and were soiling their beds. Nor was there ever enough food in the house. Three months later, in frustration, the foster-care sister turned the mother in. CYFD charged her with child abuse. The court sent her to jail and she gave up parental rights so that the children's foster parents can adopt them.

Though the kids currently live in a stable home, all the interruptions have created an emotionally damaging life for them. It's very disappointing to Deb and me. I do sometimes give in to doubts about our ability to heal infants and adults who have had trauma, or neglect, or physical or sexual abuse handed down through the generations.

What happens to the brain in the first few years affects relationships throughout our lifetime. That's why I spend so much energy searching out new ways to show parents how to support their kids. Right now Deb and I are teaching the Circle-of-Security Program to those who have lost children to the state. In eight sessions we look at parents' attachments to their own parents, as well as infants' and toddlers' developmental needs.

Q: How about an example of your success?

A: Sometimes parents just can't get their kids back, even though the goal of Infant Teams is safe reunification. But there are other types of success. The First Judicial Infant Team spent a lot of time with a woman alcoholic who was also bipolar because of early sexual abuse. Neighbors had repeatedly called 911 to say both mother and father, drunk and fighting, were endangering their four children. The police found her in the Santa Fe Place parking lot, passed out behind the wheel, with an eighteen-month-old boy strapped into his car seat in back.

The state's CYFD asked Deb and me to work with the parents during twice-a-week visits at the Early Childhood/Mental Health office over a period of nine months. The father never showed up. Even though the little boy's foster mother joined us, at first he was afraid to be in the same room with his biological mom.

After the mother got sober, Deb gave her private therapy. This included sharing videotapes taken during communal visits that showed how she looked when angry, and how her son looked when scared.

Deb and I both demonstrated ways to play with the boy, which his mom had never done, such as driving miniature cars to a play gas station to fill up, or passing a rubber ball back and forth. We also drove mother and son to a playground to swing, seesaw, and go down the slide together. Deb took photos of these joyful activities and I placed them in an album for the boy's mom to share with friends.

Because of court records showing this mother's long history of instability and alcoholism, she did not get her boy back. But she did stay sober, attended Santa Fe Community College to become a nurse's aide, and developed enough trust in Deb to talk freely about her own abuse as a child.

At the end of nine months, the mother allowed the foster parents to adopt the boy, giving her the right to negotiate for continued contact—the legal term is Open Adoption. In her case this resulted in spending two hours with him every other month, plus letters to him in between.

Q: How do you go about fund-raising?

A: The world I know is grant-writing. One grant request I sent off proposes that The Baby Fund in Santa Fe pay for Deb and me to conduct a series of seminars for teaching nurses; infant-mental-health home visitors; and speech, occupational, physical, and licensed mental-health therapists how best to work with substance-using parents and their prenatal-drug-exposed children.

My advice to readers hoping to fund a major project? Take a grant-writing class. Then spend a lot of time pinpointing the foundations sympathetic to your cause. Finally, follow each foundation's guidelines exactly.

Jane Clarke's Thumbnail Bio:

Born in Hartford, Connecticut, in 1951. MA, Our Lady of the Lake University, Jersig School of Communication Disorders, Texas, 1977. Speech/language/hearing therapist for children and their families, 1978–1993. Doctoral degree from the University of New Mexico in Special Education: Early Childhood Language/Learning Disabilities, 1993. Postgraduate work at the University of Massachusetts in Infant Mental Health. Extensive experience dealing with high-risk families, regulatory-sensory processing disorders, and prenatal alcohol-and-drug exposure. Board member of the Prajna Mountain Buddhist Order; the Step Ahead nonprofit, supporting programs that help substance-affected babies and their families heal; and, from 2007 to 2010, the New Mexican Association of Infant Mental Health.

Statistics on Birth-to-Three Mental-Health Disorders:

The term "infant mental health" implies promoting healthy social/emotional development of children from birth to three years old by increasing their ability to experience, regulate, and express emotions; to form close relationships with others; to explore the environment; and to learn. One expert, Dr. Bruce Perry, claims that 100% of children who view domestic violence develop post-traumatic stress disorder (PTSD). Over 5,000,000 infants and toddlers in this country are afflicted with PTSD, though often misdiagnosed. Children experiencing abuse or neglect are nine times more likely to become criminals, according to the US Department of Health and Human Services.

New Mexico's Children, Youth, and Families Department (CYFD) receives more than 30,000 reports of maltreatment every year.

To Help Out or Get Help:

Here are ways to access services provided by New Mexico's Children, Youth, and Families Department (CYFD):

> For general information: www.cyfd.org
> To report abuse or neglect, call (855) 333-7233
> To foster or adopt a child, call (800) 432-2075

To learn about the National Child Traumatic Stress Network, dedicated to raising the standard of care for children, their families, and their communities, log onto www.nctsn.org

Parents, early-childhood professionals, and policy-makers can find out how better to give children a strong start in life by logging onto www.zerotothree.org

To become a volunteer Court Appointed Special Advocate, named by a judge to represent the best interests of abused or neglected children in court, log onto www.casafirst.org. This is a national program.

James Serendip
High School Math Teacher

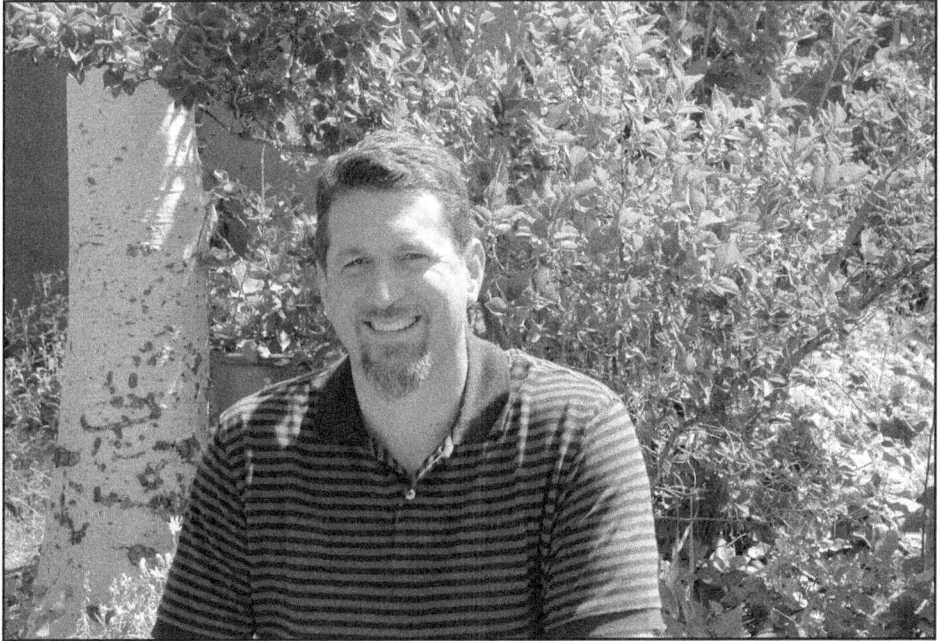

Q: James, tell us about the Academy for Technology and the Classics.

A: At the time of the publication of this book, we're three hundred and seventy students, grades seven through twelve, designated by the Santa Fe District as a charter school, meaning that, although public, we control our own budget. The only cost for attendance is an annual activities fee, in 2014 a hundred and fifty dollars.

A group of parents working at Los Alamos National Laboratory started ATC in 2000, in portable buildings near Santa Fe's Genoveva Chavez Community Center. Now our one permanent building and its basketball court sit opposite the Institute for American Indian Arts.

ATC's focus is college prep. Of our thirty-eight students who graduated in June, only two or three didn't go to college. We have roughly equal numbers of girls and boys, fifty percent Anglo, forty percent Hispanic, ten percent Asian and others. The waiting list is six hundred students long.

As of now, ours is the only high school in the Santa Fe district to receive an A grade two years in a row from New Mexico's Public Education Department. It's especially a place for kids who—too smart or too different— might not fit in at more traditional schools. Parents go online each February to sign up for ATC's lottery. Right now only twelve percent of hopefuls get in—my own daughter didn't even make it. Twelfth graders who test high on the end-of-year Advanced Placement (AP) exams sometimes can start college as sophomores.

ATC offers AP courses in English lit and comp, calculus and statistics, US and world history, physics and biology. Electives include the yearbook and our newspaper, *The Phoenix Flame*, painting and sculpture classes, and Acoustic Americana—twenty students who play roots music on guitars, violins, and banjos all over town. Calisthenics, yoga, and tai chi classes take place in the multipurpose room or cafeteria. Our sports are cross country, track and field, soccer, and basketball.

What really stands out about ATC is the students' acceptance of each other. It's far more than tolerance—they honor each others' differences. Every April fifteenth we celebrate a National Day of Silence to show solidarity with kids our culture has bullied, those with nontraditional gender identities, the disabled, and the developmentally impaired. Some of our instructors participate by teaching silently. In an afternoon ceremony that breaks that silence, students come before the whole school to share pre-ATC experience with being silenced against their wills.

Q: What are your duties at ATC?

A: Mostly I teach Advance-Placement statistics, pre-calculus, and upper-level algebra—which at ATC includes polynomial and exponential functions, logarithms, trigonometry, imaginary numbers, and matrices.

Because learning math is challenging, I try to keep the atmosphere relaxed and fun. Classes run from ten to thirty students. I spend a lot of one-on-one time getting to know them well, moving from desk to desk more than standing in front of them. Even students who answer an assignment wrong get a high grade if I can see they worked hard on the problem.

Also, I encourage them to stay authentic, not play self-defeating roles. A lot of kids come to math believing they're no good at it and ought to keep their mouths shut. I let them know that mistakes are a necessary part of learning. If someone catches me in a mistake, I give out a foam-rubber brain or a pencil with a barnyard-animal face on it. Today's kids love offbeat humor.

I like to present a lesson as a game. To speed up learning about the different kinds of numbers, I'll divide the class into two teams. They line up in front of the whiteboard where I've drawn a target with concentric rings, marking the outermost ring *real numbers*, then *rational numbers* and *integers,* with *natural numbers* written in the bull's-eye. I'll call out an example number, say "eight," and simultaneously point at a student in each team. Whoever first places a finger on *natural* gets a point. When all students have participated, the team with the most points wins. To each winning member I'll hand over a *Smartie,* a small plastic tube holding candies.

One year an eleventh grader came into my classes who had routinely failed at math. She told me she hated the subject. By the end of December she was making Cs in upper-level algebra and said she actually was enjoying herself. By the end of April, she was making Bs and asked to be considered for the Work Ethic Award. She won it. Once a year, for each class, teachers give out three awards: the Work Ethic, the Academic Excellence, and the Intellectual Curiosity awards. Parents and the student body sit in folding chairs on the basketball court while we present the certificates.

Sometimes I teach lower-level math, and occasionally tai chi. As a certified hypnotherapist, I lead workshops to deal with test anxiety, for students who want to participate and have obtained written parental consent. A group of a dozen kids and I meet six times a year to prepare for the American Math Challenge, to see how they stack up against other exceptional students around the country.

Probably I'm most famous for my waffles made from scratch, using gallons of milk and four or five dozen eggs, on the mornings of major events like the PARCC (Partnership for Assessment of Readiness for College and Careers), which students need to pass to graduate—four full days of testing. After several years at ATC, I now have twenty students, faculty, and parents who help out. Waffle irons fill the classroom. It's total chaos, eighty kids at a time. The activity breaks the stress and gets something warm into their tummies.

Q: What life experiences have contributed to your doing this good work?

A: A turning point occurred while I was earning a Master of Fine Arts in Creative Writing at the University of New Orleans. A suspicious guy had followed me home from my bartending job. Having wrapped his face in a red bandana and slipped into the unlocked duplex I was renting, he pointed a huge Glock 17 at me. I gave him whatever cash I had. He told me to lie on the floor, covered my head with my denim jacket, and shoved the end of the pistol against the back of my head. I remember thinking, *I'll never hear the shot,* but somehow made peace with what was happening. My life passed before my eyes—and I realized that all that mattered were my connections with people.

I must have fainted. When I came to, he was gone. I lay there wondering how, with the rest of my time remaining, I could be most helpful in the lives of others. Money and status no longer mattered.

Liz, whom I'd met waiting tables, and I got married, and left for Boulder, then Denver. There I wrote newsletters for seven years, offering tips to business owners until we moved to Hawaii to have our daughter. During Liz's pregnancy, we found I had a gift for guiding her into an inner, sacred space that enabled her to deliver without anesthetics. For four years in Hawaii I waited tables and worked as a carpenter and deck-hand on dive boats. We then moved to Santa Fe so that Liz's family could participate in raising Melia. Liz found a dream job as marketing manager for Nambé Mills tableware. She has a degree in industrial design.

She's the one who encouraged me to earn a certificate in hypnotherapy. I practiced for five years, gradually seeing that so many of my clients' issues began in their teenage years. I had started wishing I could work with teenagers when A+ Academic Coaching, a company in Albuquerque, hired me to use hypnosis to help its clients overcome test anxiety.

I'd decided that creative writing was too narcissistic; it had stopped serving me as therapy. As a rebel, I would never have intended to do what my dad did most of his life, teach math—statistics and algorithms—in his case at Polytechnic University on Long Island. But I picked up a lot of knowledge about the subject from him and for two years as an undergrad had studied biochemistry, which meant more math.

Soon A + Academic Coaching asked me to teach algebra and trigonometry, high school and college level both, to several of its clients. Realizing that teaching is what I loved to do, I closed my hypnotherapy practice and tried to sub all over town, in every school, grade, and subject, to see what gave me the most juice. After I'd helped out at ATC for a year, the principal offered me full-time work because the students and I got along so well. Math was the position that needed filling.

Six months later, having received a high score on the Basic Skills test, and doing well on the others, I received my Intern Teaching License from the state, good for three years. After that I earned my Alternative Teaching License.

Though I started teaching math by default, I've grown passionate about it because my greatest joy is helping people let go of limiting beliefs, exactly what I'd done using hypnosis.

Q: Any role models who inspire you?

A: Mahatma Gandhi was a lawyer but never held a political office. He died destitute yet changed the course of a nation, winning India's independence from England just by the strength of his beliefs. He proved to the world that love and peace are stronger than brute force.

My tai chi teacher when we lived in Boulder and Denver, Jane Faigao, is a constant inspiration. A small, gray-haired woman, she could, without seeming hostile, confront anyone taking the slightest shortcut. After a while she asked me to teach beginning classes. When she contracted the breast cancer that killed her, she wanted me to take over her advanced classes. I doubted my qualifications but she told me that teaching is not about being the best, it's about inspiring others to be their best.

Q: How do you arrange the rest of your life to let you do this good work?

A: Though probably I put sixty hours a week into teaching, grading, and preparing lesson plans, my wife and daughter come first. At the time of this book's publication, Melia's seventh grade schedule being the same as mine makes that a little easier. She, Liz, and I hike, walk, or run together, or just sit and talk. We try to make Sunday a family day.

Being fully present at ATC for a hundred teenagers takes a lot of energy. So I do what I can to keep fit, a half-hour of tai chi three times a week, the climbing gym once a week, shopping for and preparing non-packaged foods. I do the cooking—Liz now works as a bookkeeper for three local companies.

I love going to movies but have no time, and wish I could exercise more. Nor is there time for the elaborate dinners I used to enjoy fixing.

Q: What effect does religious or spiritual practice have on your work?

A: As a teacher, I'm not supposed to espouse religious or spiritual beliefs in the classroom, since that could make students who have different beliefs feel unsafe.

But once a year I show them videos comparing the sizes of various stars, some of them hundreds of millions of times the size of our sun. It's a way of realizing how small we are compared to what's out there. I point out that we can feel as significant as those stars since we're made of the same stuff.

The beauty of math is that it's relevant at any scale. It's the language of the universe itself. Personally, I believe that mathematics is the language of God.

I have a practice of praying out loud as I drive the twenty miles to school, asking to be fully present in the classroom so I can give the kids what they need most. Sometimes that just means being an adult who will listen, other times it's to notice who's upset and ask about it without judging, or to find the best way to explain a difficult concept like why do imaginary numbers exist. I ask for grace, not to let worries or fears interfere. I want my students to feel loved.

My two favorite rote prayers are the Serenity Prayer and one from my Episcopal upbringing that starts, "Almighty God, unto Whom all hearts are open, all desires are known...cleanse the thoughts of my heart by the inspiration of Your Holy Spirit...."

We have a number of kids who are very religious or come from religious families: Mormons, Catholics, Jews, Jehovah's Witnesses, Hindus, Buddhists. Sometimes, before school or at lunch, they like to talk about their faith or lack of it. A year ago one boy said he wanted to share why being a Jehovah's Witness didn't suit him any longer. We discussed probable consequences of leaving the faith, that neither his parents nor Jehovah Witness friends would be allowed to talk to him anymore. He couldn't stand the inner conflict and became a runaway in Chicago, but returned a year later to graduate and to reconcile with his family.

Q: What doubts and disappointments do you deal with in your work?

A: I often doubt my qualifications to be doing what I do. I don't have a degree in math or in education, yet I'm a math educator. I worry that I'm too permissive, that some students might be better served if I were more strict. Once in a while I feel that a colleague or two don't know what to make of me. I'd like to say I don't care, but that's not true.

Doubts like these motivate me to spend extra time preparing for class. I have high expectations and give the kids a lot of freedom to meet them. Occasionally a student will take advantage of that. I have caught students cheating. Those times feel like personal attacks, betrayals. After calling the parents in, I offer the student a second chance, but make it difficult. Instead of giving the test again, I'll ask for a half-hour presentation after hours, slides and a written explanation of the material. The student becomes the teacher, to experience what it's like.

My goal is transparency, to let the kids see me as a real person, so they'll trust me.

Q: More examples of your successes?

A: Let's see. Following graduation from ATC, one boy became the first in his family to get into college. He was a short, lively kid and extremely hard-working, but until coming to ATC had always struggled with math. Sometimes we butted heads. I'd show the class how to solve an equation using trigonometric identities, and he'd walk up to me at lunch to say my explanation made no sense. I told him if he'd use analytic tools that he already possessed long enough, he'd understand. It worked! He was very good at not giving up.

Some time back I got a text from him from the state university down in Las Cruces. "Hello, Mr. Serendip," he said. "I wanted to thank you for your faith in me. Yes, I gave you a hard time but you had patience.

I've just tested out of the low-math class and got put in a higher one. No words of gratitude for you are strong enough. Much love." His message made me tear up.

Then there's this gifted songwriter. Math had been a lifelong problem, but at ATC she managed to do well enough in upper-level algebra to take college-level calculus in her senior year. The University of Texas in Austin awarded her a full-ride scholarship, tuition, a travel stipend, and housing. Austin is a music town, perfect for her. She writes and sings Christian rap.

Q: How does your school go about fund-raising?

A: ATC's Parent Teacher Student Coalition—PTSC, equivalent to PTAs at other schools—runs a couple of fund-raisers. The parents also sometimes treat faculty to gourmet lunches. Last week parents brought us barbequed pork, Indian chicken curry, Thai noodles, and baked apples, which we ate on the balcony of the multipurpose room.

In early December the PTSC sells farolitos (candles, sand, and paper bags—called luminarias in much of New Mexico—to light driveways and rooftops for the holidays). We use the money to buy lab equipment. Most weekdays Real Burger brings in student lunches, but every other Friday PTSC sells pizza. The proceeds go towards funding school events.

Students pay twenty-five dollars to participate in our early October, five-kilometer Flaming Chicken Run; ATC's mascot is the phoenix. There's also the Albertson's Community Partners key-chain card. One percent of your grocery bill goes back to ATC. If you buy products from Amazon, you can request that up to six percent, depending on the item, be sent to ATC. Any item showing the BoxTops for Education logo—cereals, snacks, Ziploc bags, purchases from retailers like Land's End and Walmart—can help us. Just turn in the box tops to ATC's front office.

A Santa-Fe-only charity, connecting teachers with donors, is

Dollars4Schools.org. I'm writing a grant request for a thousand dollars to buy five hard-copy, college-level statistics texts. They should stay relevant for maybe ten years. If I bought the online version, the seventy-dollar license to use it would need renewing every year.

James Serendip's Thumbnail Bio:

Born on Long Island, New York, 1970. BA Philosophy and Creative Writing, State University of New York at Binghampton. MFA Creative Writing, University of New Orleans. Wrote newsletters in Boulder and Denver offering tips to business owners, 1995–2002. Waited tables and worked as carpenter and deckhand in Kona, HI, 2002–2006. Certified hypnotherapist in Santa Fe, 2007–2011. Substitute teacher in Santa Fe, 2011–2012. Full-time math teacher, grades 7-12, at The Academy for Technology and the Classics, 2012–present.

Statistics on US High School Math Performance:

In 2014, results from the federally funded National Assessment of Educational Progress, aka The Nation's Report Card, showed that only 26% of students in fourth, eighth, and twelfth grades scored at or above proficient in math, no different than the results in 2009, slightly above results in 2005. Asian, Pacific Islander, and White students scored higher than Hispanic, American Indian, and Black students. Approximately 47,000 students participated in the study.

In 2013, only 44% of US high school graduates were prepared for college math. In 2012, high school students in 26 industrialized nations performed better in math than their US counterparts. High school students who complete at least upper-level algebra are twice as likely to win a college degree as those who do not.

To Help Out, or Get Help:

The Academy for Technology and the Classics
    74 A Van Nu Po
    Santa Fe, NM 87508
    (505) 473-4282
    www.atcschool.org

    www.dayofsilence.org
    (national organization honoring gay, lesbian, and straight students)

    www.khanacademy.org
    (instructional videos in math and physics)   (continued)

www.donorschoose.org
(national online charity for public schools)

www.dollars4schools.org
(Santa Fe online charity)

Talitha Arnold
Senior Minister, United Church of Santa Fe

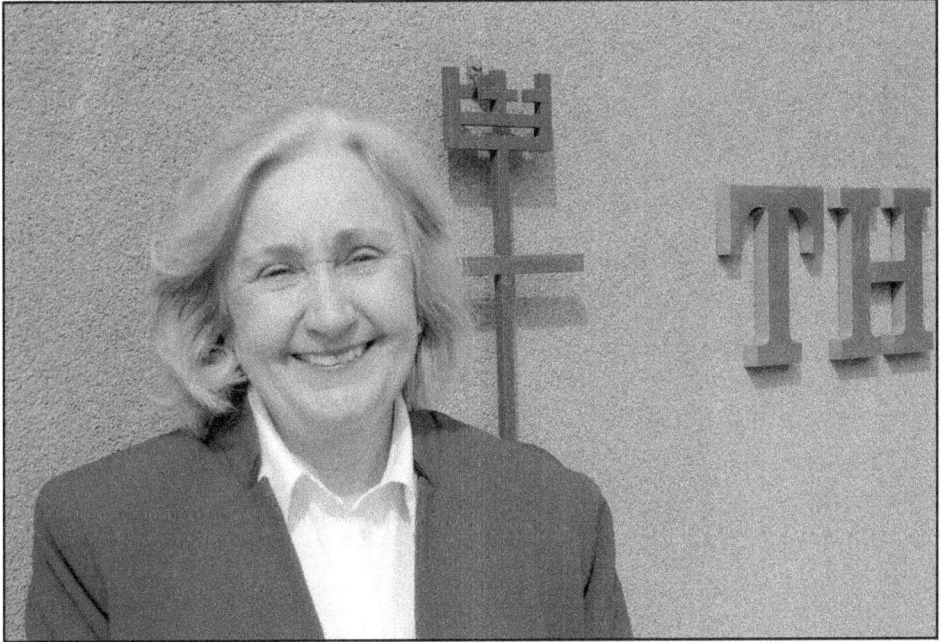

Q: Talitha, tell us about your church and your role there.

A: The church started in Santa Fe in the bar at El Gancho in 1980. Founding Minister Reverend Martha Baumer was soon able to move the congregation of about thirty to the music room of St. Michael's High. We are part of the nationwide group, United Church of Christ, not to be confused with the more conservative Church of Christ in the South and Southwest.

The congregation asked me to be its pastor in 1987. Today we sit on three and a half acres catercorner from the hospital. Eighty percent of our four hundred parishioners are Anglo; ten to fifteen percent are Hispanic.

Half of our children are adopted—Mexican, Guatemalan, Southern Indian, South Korean, Chinese, African, and Native American.

Not tumbleweed hope but deep-rooted, piñon hope is at the heart of what I do. We believe that Christ, an incarnation of the Mystery that moves the universe, died not to save us from our sins, but *because* of the sins of injustice and the abuse of power. Worship is meant to provide an experience of God's love, impelling us to go out into the world and love it as God does.

Caring for others takes up a big part of my day. A few years ago the grandson of a couple who'd been members when I arrived told me his sister had died of an overdose of heroin in Cleveland, Ohio. But his parents wanted services held in Santa Fe. They needed a community that would be there for them. So we created a memorial service for them here.

Many of the students in Santa Fe's public schools seem to live at the poverty level. In the mid-nineties, the principal at an elementary school, one of our members, gave a presentation at our morning forum on education. A retired couple from Chicago—who'd owned a string of auto-mechanic schools in Detroit—wanted to help. They mustered volunteers to assist in classrooms and tutor individually. In ten years the group grew from five to thirty-five, transitioning to become a branch of a national organization called Communities in Schools.

We put a lot of energy into social-justice issues—mental health, poverty, homelessness, care for the environment, immigration, gender equality. I've been doing same-gender marriages since 1989, not officially legal in New Mexico until 2013, but blessed in the eyes of the church. In 2014, the Associate Minister and I did at least a hundred same-gender weddings, including two men who had adopted a son a decade prior.

Writing and public speaking are central to my ministry. At least once a year I testify at the state legislature on issues like gun violence and environmental concerns, and submit op-ed pieces to *The New Mexican*. Often ideas for sermons come from these efforts, and vice versa. Every Sunday I face a congregation of hundred and fifty editors. When I see someone nodding, or eyes rolling back, or checking a watch, I know that's where I need to cut.

When I became pastor, the church had no secretary, pianist, children's minister, or custodian. We were paying sixty-five thousand dollars a year on a half-million-dollar mortgage. In 1995 we burned that mortgage, took on another in 1998 to expand the buildings, and have almost reduced that one to nothing. Today we pay the following full-time employees: our office administrator, a family and community director, and a pastoral intern. Paid, part-time staff include our pianist/music director, children's choir director, adult choir director, children's ministry director, teachers, a child care provider, a custodian, and a contract CPA. Volunteers provide the lion's share of what needs doing, from keeping up the grounds to pastoral and child care, mentoring youth, and meals for the homeless.

I myself put in sixty to seventy hours a week. A good image for ministry is the little man in the circus who spins plates. His goal is to get ten plates spinning, but when he succeeds with six or seven, plate number one starts to drop.

Q: What life experiences have contributed to your doing this good work?

A: My father, who'd been a lieutenant on a minesweeper in the North Pacific, came out of World War II with what was called shell shock or battle fatigue—the term post-tramatic stress disorder hadn't been invented. As a biologist for the Fish and Wildlife Service, he took up research on golden and bald eagles, convinced the bounty on them should be removed. But lobbyists for the ranchers stopped his findings from getting published.

Like my father, whom I never met, my mother also had a master's. Hers was in microbiology. During the war she'd done research for Cutter Labs in how best to mass-produce penicillin. Infections were killing more of our soldiers than bullets or bombs.

By 1953, both parents were living on a national wildlife refuge in the northeast corner of California. My brothers were six and seven, my sister was four, Mother was three months pregnant with me. My father flew to Washington DC so that he could plead the eagles' case with the Secretary of the Interior. There he had a breakdown, and was committed to Saint Elizabeth's Hospital, where he stayed until the Veterans Administration transferred him to another mental hospital in San Diego. Two years later, out on a three-day pass, he bought a handgun and took his life.

When he was hospitalized in DC, Mother and my siblings flew to South Phoenix to move in with her mother because they had nowhere else to go. Mother had no car. So though she and my father had been participating Episcopalians, she returned to the faith of her childhood and took us to the nearby Congregational church, now part of the United Church of Christ.

Ecology and issues of mental health have long been deep concerns of mine. But having grown up in a Christian community is key to what I do. I've always been interested in the Mystery. The great Bible stories like Noah's Ark and David and Goliath captivated me. At church potlucks I loved the tuna casseroles and chocolate cake, basic comfort food. I also loved singing in the children's choir, making baskets in Sunday school, and fixing typical Biblical food like unleavened bread.

Mostly I gained confidence from the kids and adults around me that we were capable of helping others. We collected canned goods for people in need, and wrote birthday cards to the sick and homebound.

After my birth in Phoenix, Mother started a twenty-five-year career of teaching science in middle school, to keep to the same schedule as my siblings. No matter how late she went to bed, she'd begin each day by reading the Bible and a devotional text. Her tenacity and deep-rooted faith kept us all going. My sister is now a veterinarian surgeon, one brother is an environmental lawyer, the other is a personal injury lawyer. We're each a minister, I feel, following callings to make this world a better place.

Personally and as a pastor, I've experienced what I call 'Christ events.' I don't mean a flash of light or Hallelujah Chorus, I mean coming to a dead end and reconnecting to life in a new way. One of the most powerful occurred when I was twenty-five and serving as Associate Minister at the First Congregational Church in Tempe, Arizona. I'd been involved for five years with a guy I'd met at Pomona College. He was in Tahiti on a fellowship, trying to do in photographs what Gauguin had done in paint. Though I think really he was studying Tahitian men, because when I flew over to visit him, he announced he was gay.

I certainly supported gay rights. Yet as his girlfriend, what was I supposed to do with that information? I kept quiet; this was 1978. But many of my parishioners, having survived into their sixties and seventies, provided examples of how to live through dead ends, stay open to new life.

Q: Any role models who inspire you?

A: The African-American Reverend Doctor Reuben A. Sheares III is one. In a predominantly white environment, he headed up the United Church of Christ's New York based Office for Church Life and Leadership in the nineteen-eighties. Slight of stature physically, he was tall in other ways, having the courage often to be the only African-American in the room. He had large hands, a big smile on a broad, clean-shaven face, and always wore a suit and tie. He'd grown up in South Carolina in the years of Jim Crow segregation.

This man lived by several precepts that helped me mature as a leader: to stay focused on the goals of the church, to be sure all voices of leadership are heard, not to be afraid to make hard decisions, and to remember that coming together for worship and prayer empowers every-thing else we do.

Reuben was a preacher from his toes up, making ancient stories relevant. He showed, for instance, how doubting Thomas—John, chapter 20—was actually the most faithful of the disciples. John demonstrates that the resurrected Christ is known not only in glory but also by his wounds, representing the wounds of this world.

My current role models are the members of our church. They believe in the parable of the Last Judgment, ending Matthew 25. Those who feed the hungry, visit the sick, welcome the stranger, clothe the naked, and comfort the prisoner truly see the face of God. It's the heart of the Gospel for us.

When we see an end coming, as Christ did at the Last Supper, we summon the fortitude to embrace new beginnings. I recall a couple of parishioners with sons eight and eleven. Two weeks before Christmas the father died at the hands of a drunk driver. After grieving for two years, the mother found a full-time job teaching college-level art history, to save funds for putting the boys through college. She resumed singing in the church choir—I can still see her singing the "Hallelujah Chorus" at Easter with tears streaming down her face. For the church, she created an adult-ed class, "The Feminine Face of God," with art going back thirty-eight thousand years.

Q: How do you arrange the rest of your life to let you do this good work?

A: Sometimes I don't sleep a lot. I try to nurture a sense of humor about myself and others. I look up at the mountains, trees, and sky as often as I can. After waking at six, I skip breakfast except for a cup of coffee, then walk Nizhoni, a stray reservation dog whose name is Navajo for 'beauty', around the neighborhood. Sometimes I'll read or clean house until driving to church before eight.

A pastor's work is not neat and tidy; you do what the day demands and try to keep your hair combed. Lunches are often in a restaurant, trading ideas with members of the congregation or meeting someone from the wider community to talk about issues like poverty or public education.

Typically I get back home between eight-thirty and nine. Meals are a challenge of being single—by the age of ten I was the main chef for my mother and three siblings. I don't enjoy cooking for myself. Dinner on good days may be take-home chicken and a salad, on bad days chocolate-chip cookies I've scrounged from the church kitchen. I'm afraid the vegans reading this will say, "I don't want to go to that church, the pastor has poor eating habits."

After dinner I'll sometimes do *The New York Times* crossword puzzle to help me sleep. In bed I look back over the day and think of ten things I'm thankful for. Then, over and over, I breathe in God's peace, God's hope, and God's deep, abiding love, just as I invite parishioners to do.

Music is important in our church and a big part of my life elsewhere. From September to May I sing alto in the Santa Fe Symphony Chorus. And I'm trying to carve out time for rejoining the week-long Berkshire Choral Festival. One hundred and fifty of us have sung in Santa Fe, the California wine country, Massachusetts, Austria, and the Czech Republic.

I've hiked the Grand Canyon several times, and been able to raft it twice, thanks to friends. In 2014 I hiked around the Judean Desert, as well as the forty-mile-long Jesus Trail from Nazareth to the Sea of Galilee. In January 2015, a friend and I got our Sonoran Desert cactus fix, five days in Sedona and Phoenix.

Q: How do you shape your sermons for maximum effect?

A: The challenge of preaching is that your text is at least two thousand years old, separated from the congregation by time, ethnicity, geography, and culture. My joy is to show how that text speaks to us who live in a much different world.

My sermons are about fifteen minutes long. I hope they'll do two things, connect the congregation to the Mystery we call God, and help parishioners realize that we're dealing with the same issues as the ancients: how to find new life after hitting a dead end; how to include more people as neighbors and care for them; how to find wisdom in a complicated world; and how to open our eyes, ears, and lives to the presence of God in ourselves and in everything else.

This past Sunday I based a sermon, "Connected to Courage," on chapter 1 of Ruth, where Naomi walks forward after losing her husband

and two sons. A sermon before that, "Connected to All Creation," took its cue from Psalm 104, affirming God's presence everywhere.

Based on a theme, I plan a series of sermons three months in advance, and write out each a week ahead. This gives me time for revisions. I'll even revise between speaking to the eight-thirty and the later-morning congregations, depending on their response or how their demographics differ. One of my sermons dealt with the Nativity story. Since not many parents attend the early service, for that one I focused on the shepherds and the innkeeper. For the later service, I emphasized how Mary must have felt carrying a child, and how Joseph must have wondered about parenting a child not his own.

The opening sentence has to be a grabber, such as "The rosebush had no business being there," which I used recently, referring to Isaiah's vision of a desert in bloom. I try to flesh out each story with details to make it live. Mark 9, verses 2 through 8, tells of Jesus taking three disciples up a high mountain where God transfigured Him into a glorious image of light. I started the sermon by having the congregation imagine how hot, sweaty, dirty, and stinky that hike must have been.

Years ago I started emailing a five-hundred-word synopsis of each sermon to the entire congregation on the Friday prior. Not only does that discipline me, but it gives the congregation a head start on imagining the story I'll be using in worship.

Q: What doubts and disappointments do you deal with in your work?

A: This country's consumer culture permeates our spirituality. So many people speak of "church shopping, synagogue shopping," asking how a particular community of faith meets their needs. Shouldn't they also be seeking a form of worship that glorifies God? Doesn't having a spiritual life mean focusing on the needs of others as well as one's own?

A big doubt I have is wondering what difference I'm making. It's like teaching—there's no tangible product except people. Oscar Romero, the archbishop in El Salvador, killed by a death squad in 1980, said,

"We're called to be ministers, not messiahs. We plant seeds for others to harvest." This helps me do what I can, without expecting to change the world.

Every preacher occasionally suffers the dark night of the soul, when the internal well goes dry and God is silent. My darkest nights are when I come up against limits of compassion and understanding. In those times I acknowledge how I'm feeling, then read about others wrenched by similar experiences. Or go for a walk while consciously breathing in God's gifts of courage, patience, and hope, even if at the moment they're hard to access. And I seek out friends.

As the head of staff, I never know what surprises are coming down the pike. In a six-month period we had a child-care provider move to Guam to be near family, an associate minister move to Oklahoma and our choral director to Alabama, both for new jobs.

Many people seem to use Santa Fe as a way station. The retired come here for the arts and beautiful sunsets, then ten years later leave to be closer to relatives or return to lower altitudes. The young go away after discovering our high cost of living or lack of job opportunities. So you work, work, work to build a church community and, like the Red Queen in *Through the Looking-Glass*, run, run, run just to stay in place.

There's always the disappointment that neither the church nor I can be all things to all people. Within a few years after I came on board here, the majority of the congregation voted to be 'open and affirming' in welcoming the LGBT (Lesbian, Gay, Bisexual, and Transgender) community. The change in acceptance took two years. Some parishioners who disagreed left. Others left because we hadn't moved fast enough.

Six years later, we expanded the sanctuary from a hundred to two hundred and seventy chairs, changing from a family-style church to a larger, more diverse population that could do a lot more good works. Some members who liked the smaller church left. Others adjusted. The analogy is the family that adds more children. Often the older siblings get upset. As the youngest of four, I know that first hand. Of course, I gave them a lot to be upset about!

Q: Will you share more examples of your successes?

A: Our main success is growing from a struggling congregation of ninety in the early nineteen-eighties to over four hundred today. The financial support we give organizations that house the homeless, feed the hungry, educate children, and care for the environment has quadrupled in twenty years. Just as important are the members of our congregation, a couple of hundred at least, who volunteer their time to good works.

Take serving Santa Fe's homeless. Nearly twenty of our parishioners once a month cook dinners at home and bring them to the men at St. Elizabeth Shelter. Half a dozen of our teenagers go there monthly to clean bathrooms, sort cabinets, or decorate for holidays. A third group cooks dinners for the single women and families with children at St. Elizabeth's Casa Familia. Sixty other volunteers put in a week at the Interfaith Community Shelter, bringing in meals and welcoming guests for the night. Another dozen of us lobby the city council and state legislature for more-humane laws and greater funding for affordable housing.

Q: How do you go about fund-raising?

A: We feel that caring for those in need should represent the first fruits of the harvest. Percentage-giving makes clear how much you're spending on others, compared to spending on yourself.

Fund-raising is far more than technique. It's about vision—understanding and communicating the purpose of an organization. It's also about leading by example. For instance, I tithe ten percent of my salary to the church. That's in addition to supporting refugee relief, Pomona College, Yale Divinity School, the National Parks Association, and the Santa Fe Symphony. I can't ask anyone else to do what I'm not willing to do.

Nine-tenths of our budget comes from annual pledges. The drive runs from mid-October to early November, when we host a simple catered dinner. About two hundred attend. A pledge card sits at every place setting. We're an alcohol-free church, to show people how to have a good time without drinking, to support members in recovery, and because we don't want the liability. At the dinner we sing sacred songs from around the world, the children's choir sings, and three or four of our lay leaders explain why they pledge.

We also hold fund-raisers for outreach organizations. Not only does this provide them with money but publicity, too. By advertising these events citywide, we invite all to participate.

Each May we sponsor a 5K run, called United We Run, starting at the church and down St. Michaels into the arroyo. The proceeds go to three groups, different every spring. In 2015 New Mexico's Conservation Trust had to do with the environment, United Way's First Born with infant care, and Youth Emergency Shelter with homelessness.

Early in December we organize Compassionate Christmas Gifts, asking Santa Feans to buy a present for ten to fifty dollars. A Church World Service Hygiene Kit for refugee relief costs ten dollars. A backback holding a teddy bear, pajamas, a toothbrush, and a water bottle—for a child at the Solace Crisis Treatment Center—costs twenty dollars. These are just two of nine options.

Talitha Arnold's Thumbnail Bio:

Born in Phoenix, Arizona, 1953. Double BA cum laude, Religious Studies and Political Science, Pomona College, California, 1975. MDiv Yale Divinity School, Connecticut, 1980. Associate Chaplain, Yale University, 1980–1981. Associate Minister, First Church (United Church of Christ), Middletown, Connecticut, 1981–1987. Senior Minister, United Church of Santa Fe, 1987–present. President, Habitat for Humanity in Santa Fe, 1992–1994. Member, Christus St. Vincent Regional Medical Center Ethics Committee, 2006–present. Co-leader, Faith Communities Task Force, National Action Alliance for Suicide Prevention, 2010–present. Awards: Yale Divinity School's Outstanding Recent Alum, 1996; United Church of Christ's Antoinette Brown Award for outstanding women clergy, 2007; Santa Fe's *The Santa Fe New Mexican*'s Ten Who Made a Difference award, 2010. Author of *Worship for Vital Congregations*, Pilgrim Press, 2006. In progress: *A Desert Faith for a Desert Time.*

Statistics on Christian Churches:

There are 350,000 Christian congregations and approximately 247,000,000 Christian parishioners in America; on any given Sunday, 118,000 of these attend services. A congregation's average size is 75 people. Ten percent of Christian ministers are women.

The United Church of Christ has 5,300 congregations and 1,100,000 parishioners.

To Find Out More:

International

> World Council of Churches
> Route de Ferney 150
> Geneva, Switzerland
> www.oikoumene.org

National

National Council of Churches
110 Maryland Avenue NE
Suite 108
Washington, DC 20002-5603
(202) 544-2350
www.nationalcouncilofchurches.us
info@nationalcouncilofchurches.us

United Church of Christ headquarters
700 Prospect Avenue East
Cleveland, OH 44115
(216) 736-2100
www.ucc.org

In Santa Fe

United Church of Santa Fe
1808 Arroyo Chamisa Road
Santa Fe, NM 87505
(505) 988-3295
www.unitedchurchofsantafe.org
unitedchurch.talitha@gmail.com

Kim Straus
Manager, Brindle Foundation

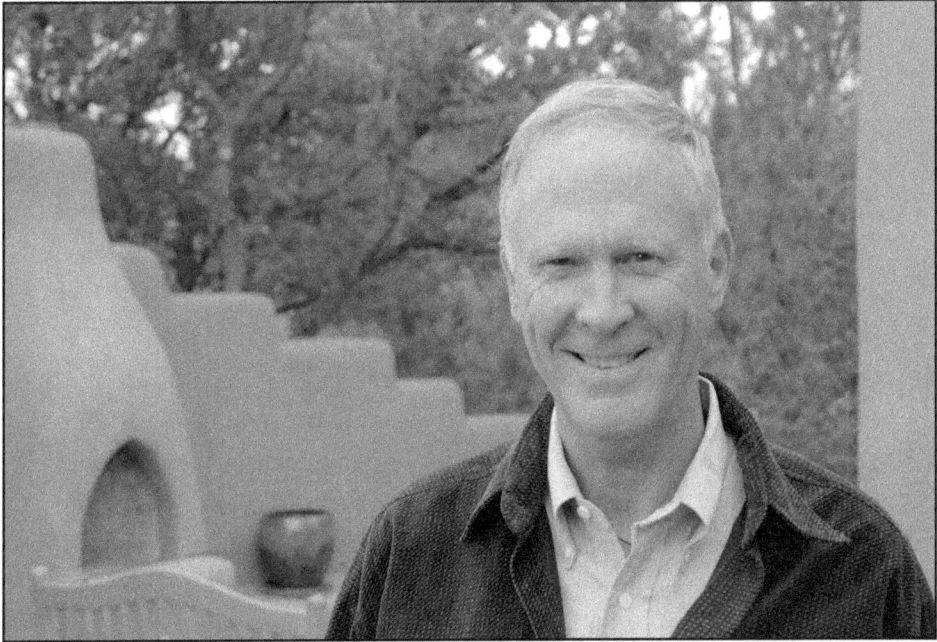

Q: Tell us about the foundation and your duties there, Kim.

A: We fund over fifty organizations in New Mexico that help babies thrive—having learned that eighty-five percent of brain development occurs by the age of three. Nan Schwanfelder, our current president, named the foundation Brindle in 2002 after her beloved, black-and-white Labrador retriever.

In 1900 Nan's great-grandfather started Utah Construction Company, a builder of dams like the O'Shaughnessy in Yosemite and Hoover Dam. When the company merged with General Electric sixty years later, it was worth 478 million dollars. Around thirty million of that is now Brindle's, allowing us to give away a little over a million dollars each year.

Nan and her two sons oversee the investments and award grants that range from ten thousand dollars for first-time grantees to forty thousand dollars. Some grantees, such as the Court-Appointed Special Advocates, Las Cumbres Community Services' Infant Program, and Food Depot have been with us for ten years.

As an example of how we decide to fund, let's take the First Born Program of Northern New Mexico, which provides home-based services to first-time parents in San Miguel and Mora counties. Its staff visits homes every week for up to three years. Only three to four percent of New Mexican families are currently getting such services. A First Born paraprofessional may bring books and ask the mother to read to her baby every day, starting before birth if possible. Or the home visitor may ask, "Are your breasts sore? Is the baby latching on?" explaining why breast-feeding builds a child's immune system better than formula.

A year and a half ago, First Born's program manager took Nan and me on a heart-wrenching visit. Because mom was in prison for dealing meth, and dad had disappeared, the baby lived with the aunt, overweight and having trouble getting around. Soon after our trip, I emailed the manager, requesting a single-page proposal and budget; all current potential grantees first submit a letter of intent.

Now a First Born home visitor accompanies the aunt to the supermarket, offers relief time, and makes sure the baby gets to doctors' appointments. Although the grandmother lives close by, she is a heroin addict and unavailable. You can imagine the aunt's gratitude for First Born.

Since we award all grants at year's end, proposals must be in by fall. So most of Nan's and my twenty-five or thirty site visits take place in September and October. Because we love to feed people, we also schedule lunches close to our headquarters.

I represent the foundation on two statewide planning groups, Early Childhood Comprehensive Systems and the New Mexico Act-Early

Team. The first advises the New Mexico Department of Health, the second advises the Center for Development and Disability at UNM (University of New Mexico). We want to expand screening for motor skills, as well as social and emotional development. The forms that accomplish this ask questions like, "Is your toddler able to grasp a toy? Is he babbling at the right age?" To a pediatrician or pediatric nurse, the answers can give an early warning of autism, for instance.

I'm also proud of being part of New Mexico's J. Paul Taylor Early Childhood Task Force, a forum of thirty early-childhood advocates who meet monthly at UNM. Our twenty-page report advises the state legislature each January how best to help youngsters at high risk—those with alcohol- or drug-affected parents, undocumented parents, jobless or homeless parents, single parents, violent parents. We've recommended that all insurance companies switch to an identical health-risk-assessment questionnaire, and include queries such as "Did you have an alcoholic mother or father? Were you abused as a young child?"

Q: What life experiences have contributed to your doing this good work?

A: My mother, who died at age one hundred and two, was a consummate volunteer and leader—president of the board of Houston's Planned Parenthood, national board member of United Way. After moving to Santa Fe in 1995, I was offered two jobs: to raise funds at Cornerstones for architectural preservation, or to serve as an administrative assistant for the New Mexico Community Foundation. I asked my mother for advice. She then asked me, "Which has the most risk?" By that she meant the most challenges and greatest opportunity to make a difference. Best advice I ever got.

I've always loved the outdoors and fine art. Between the ages of ten and fourteen, I spent summers at Cimarroncita Ranch Camp north of Taos, hiking, learning to ride, crafting silver jewelry, making mobiles from the rusted parts of tractors and old cars. I loved that camp so much that

I became a junior counselor, then counselor, then assistant director of the boys' camp, then director at age twenty-three—the girls' camp was on the other side of the hill. I developed a love for New Mexico's natural beauty and well-rooted American Indian and Hispanic cultures. I also saw that children under stress back home, whose parents might be divorcing, could learn in the great outdoors to feel safe and be their enthusiastic, energetic selves. In other words, be kids.

I realized that working in philanthropy could make a huge impact on the lives of New Mexico's children.

Q: Any current or recent role models who inspire you?

A: Nan Schwanfelder is one of the wisest people I've met. She's especially adept at knowing when we should give money for core operations rather than for a specific project simply because it's sexy. If a nonprofit proposed funding toddlers learning how to make adobe bricks, for instance, Nan might say, "That seems more appropriate for teens or adults, but we may want to help keep you financially strong."

Nan's older son was late in talking. Her younger son has dyslexia. She had the means to pay for their special education, but before starting Brindle, said to me, "What do people do who have no money, or no clue about how to advocate for their children?"

Another role model is Angie Vachio. She cofounded Albuquerque's Peanut Butter and Jelly Family Services in 1972. The organization serves more than a thousand families in Bernalillo and Sandoval counties. It runs a preschool, provides therapists for children with developmental problems, works with parents in prison, and, like First Born, sends staff to the homes of first-time mothers and fathers.

Angie and her husband have retired to a coffee plantation in Costa Rica. While she was active, she did a lot of advocating with legislators and state agencies. She knew what at-risk families need: compassion, and to be recognized for their strengths, not their weaknesses.

Q: How do you arrange the rest of your life to let you do this good work?

A: I have a husband, Jack, and, at the time this book was published, an eleven-year-old son from Guatemala, José. They respect what I do for Brindle. And in Nan Schwanfelder I have a boss who's really flexible, giving me time for family.

Jack and I have been together since 2000, officially married in 2013. I think he'd agree that our greatest achievement is being dads. As principal at El Camino Real Academy—825 kids, grades pre-K through eight, the third largest public school in the district—Jack has a workweek even longer than mine, so mostly I'm the one who drives José to piano and Spanish lessons once a week. We take turns cooking but Jack buys groceries and actually enjoys cleaning house.

We have a cabin in the Sangre de Cristo mountains an hour west of Santa Fe where the three of us sometimes spend weekends, though mostly we're regulars at the United Church of Santa Fe. José sings in the children's choir, Jack serves on the Youth Committee, and I'm on the Outreach Committee, bringing food to the homeless at the Interfaith Shelter, for example.

Jack, José, and I love to travel, twice a year on weeklong church-sponsored trips, for two to four weeks abroad in the summer. We've been to India, Peru, Mexico, Hawaii, and most recently, Tanzania in East Africa.

My independent activities include serving as copresident of the PTA at José's school, Chaparral Elementary, leading tours of Randall Davey's home and studio at the Audubon Center and Sanctuary, and volunteering in July at the Folk Art Market up on Museum Hill. I also love to turn out wood furniture and sculptures of wood and found objects from my shop in the garage.

Q: What effect does religious or spiritual practice have on your work?

A: I think it has little effect. I'm involved with church because I like the people, I respect its liberal values, and because Jack and I want to give José a chance to decide if he wants to continue to make church-going a part of his life. On Sunday mornings I pray but otherwise not, nor do I meditate.

My father was Jewish. As a child in Wisconsin, my mother went to a Presbyterian or Episcopal church, whichever happened to be convenient. Religion in our family just wasn't that important. I'm not atheistic because I admit there may be forces beyond our reasoning. I don't believe, however, that human beings are better than other creatures. I marvel at human creativity, but shrink from the devastating conflicts started in the name of religion.

Q: What doubts and disappointments do you deal with in your work?

A: A major disappointment is that many legislators don't see the cost-effectiveness of funding early-childhood programs. New Mexico spends ten times more—over $400 million every year—on prisons, juvenile justice, and child protection, than on helping babies thrive while their brains are developing. You can't protect an infant by punishing the abuser, except to stop further harm. The damage has been done. Supporting babies and their families means the child will be ready for school, less likely to break the law or become a teen parent, and more likely to finish high school, find meaningful employment, and give back to the community.

A personal worry is that, as a grant-maker, I become too pigheaded. I wish more often I could just shut up. When I was chairing the J. Paul Taylor Early Childhood Task Force, a pediatrician from the hospital at the University of New Mexico asked us to endorse the hospital's efforts to get two million dollars to treat abused infants, before she requested the money from the legislature. I don't recall if we made that endorsement or not. I remember only my chagrin at arguing that it might be better to spend money on services helping families under stress. Later I felt arrogant, that I hadn't respected her experience. She's the one who has to treat these battered children.

Nan shares with me another disappointment. Our foundation

doesn't have enough resources to fund everyone doing great work for youngsters in this state. It's emotionally hard for us to say no.

Q: How about some examples of your successes?

A: A local author for teens, Diane Stanley, brought us an idea from San Antonio: the hospitals there give a first book to every baby delivered.

I took on the task of creating Books for Babies New Mexico. Friends of the Santa Fe Public Library, head librarian Pat Hodapp, the Santa Fe Institute, and St. Vincent Hospital Foundation helped us get started. Students at Santa Fe University of Art and Design created the jackrabbit logo and brochure. Local businesses printed it and imprinted the diaper bags with *I Read To My Baby Every Day*. When parents pick up their infant's birth certificate, their bright yellow diaper bag comes with a book—*Goodnight Moon* is the most popular. The bag also contains the brochure explaining why early reading is so important for bonding, as well as for healthy brain development. It contains a CD of lullabies funded by the Santa Fe Maternal and Child Health Council and the New Mexico Department of Health, and an application for a library card.

In 2015, two years after the launch, St. Vincent gave away sixteen hundred bags. And a second hospital joined up, Socorro General Hospital. Although Brindle provided start-up funding of forty-five thousand dollars, Santa Fe's St. Vincent Hospital Foundation keeps the program going.

Another Brindle-inspired success is Diaper Depot, now part of Santa Fe's The Food Depot, presently headed by Sherry Hooper. Nan had heard about a diaper bank in Washington DC, and we discovered more than a hundred around the country. Research shows that some parents cut back on food or utilities to afford disposable diapers, thus allowing them to hold a job after dropping their babies off at child care—for sanitary reasons, no child-care facility will allow the use of cloth diapers. Other parents leave children in soiled diapers longer than they should. Some even resort to cleaning out or drying dirty diapers. So many Americans don't know this problem exists. Clean diapers are as important to a baby's well being as food and shelter.

The Food Depot supplies one hundred and thirty-five partner agencies throughout Northern New Mexico: homeless shelters, youth programs, church-based food distribution programs, senior centers, homes for the mentally disabled, shelters for battered families. In 2012 Brindle's five thousand dollar planning grant allowed the organization to do a citywide drive, setting up bins outside grocery stores. Volunteers, including Nan and me—such fun!—asked shoppers to buy disposable diapers and drop them in the bins. Now Diaper Depot also provides partner agencies with sanitary wipes, baby powder and lotion, baby food, and formula for mothers who can't breast-feed. We've continued with the grants every year—in 2015, thirty thousand dollars.

Parties are also a good way to collect disposable diapers. My husband Jack once threw me a birthday surprise party. For presents, he asked everybody to bring a box of diapers. Fifty to sixty friends came. One who couldn't, having become ill, carried that box of diapers in his car for two years until remembering to give it to me.

Q: How do you and Nan Schwanfelder decide whom to fund?

A: The quick answer is, we look for heart. That means passion, commitment, and competence. When we're investing in an organization, we're really investing in people.

Fund-raising is an art. I always say to someone trying to raise money, "Every *No* puts you closer to *Yes*. Of course you fear rejection when you ask for money. But each time you ask, you become better able to convey what your organization is best at. Chances are you won't receive a donation if you don't ask." I also say, "You'll be more successful at raising funds by knowing which foundations to approach. Do your research." You'd be amazed at how many misguided requests for funds we get from people who haven't learned that Brindle focuses on early-childhood programs.

Just as babies need nurturing relationships with their mothers to thrive, recipients of funds need to develop bonds with their donors. This takes time, thoughtfulness, and patience. Send a thank-you note to your donors. Learn what a donor's passions are. And stay true to your mission. Don't bend it just to attract more donors. Savvy donors can see through that.

Kim Straus's Thumbnail Bio:

Born in Houston, Texas, in 1953. AB from Kenyon College, Ohio, 1976. EdM in Education Administration from Harvard University, 1990. Undergraduate admissions officer, sequentially, at Kenyon College, College of Santa Fe, Lawrence University, WI, 1981–1995. Manager, Brindle Foundation, 2002–present. Co-chair, Santa Fe County Maternal & Child Health Planning Council, 2008–2012. Board member, New Mexico Childrens' Trust Fund, 2010–2013. Member, J. Paul Taylor Early Childhood Task Force, 2013–present. Member, Santa Fe County Health Planning and Policy Commission, and Santa Fe Mayor's Children, Youth and Families Community Cabinet, 2015–present. Father with husband Jack of adopted son from Guatemala.

Statistics on Young Children at Risk:

New Mexico has the highest rate of child poverty in the country, 30% compared with 23% nationally. Other at-risk indicators are children attending preschool: 41% NM, 48% US. Children in single-parent families: 38% NM, 31% US. Children in families where household head lacks a high-school diploma: 15% NM, 12% US. Source: *2015 Kids Count*, New Mexico Voices for Children.

According to the federal Substance Abuse and Mental Health Services Administration, 20% of New Mexico's adults had experienced physical abuse as a child, 13% had experienced sexual abuse, 30% had lived with a household member who abused substances, and 19% had lived with a mentally ill household member and/or witnessed domestic violence in their home. Adverse experiences like these can not only predict health outcomes later in life such as depression and heart problems, they also put the children in the care of these adults at risk.

To Find Out More:

Brindle Foundation
PO Box 31619
Santa Fe, NM 87594-1696
(505) 986-3983
www.brindlefoundation.org
kim@brindlefoundation.org

www.zerotothree.org/ offers parents and caregivers best ways to improve a child's development during the critical first thousand days of life.

www.ed.gov/early-learning/talk-read-sing enriches a child's language experience from birth on.

www.families.naeyc.org. Positive guidance from the National Association for the Education of Young Children (infants, toddlers, preschoolers).

www.nmvoices.org compares data about children in New Mexico with data nationwide.

Barbara Rockman
Poet, Teacher

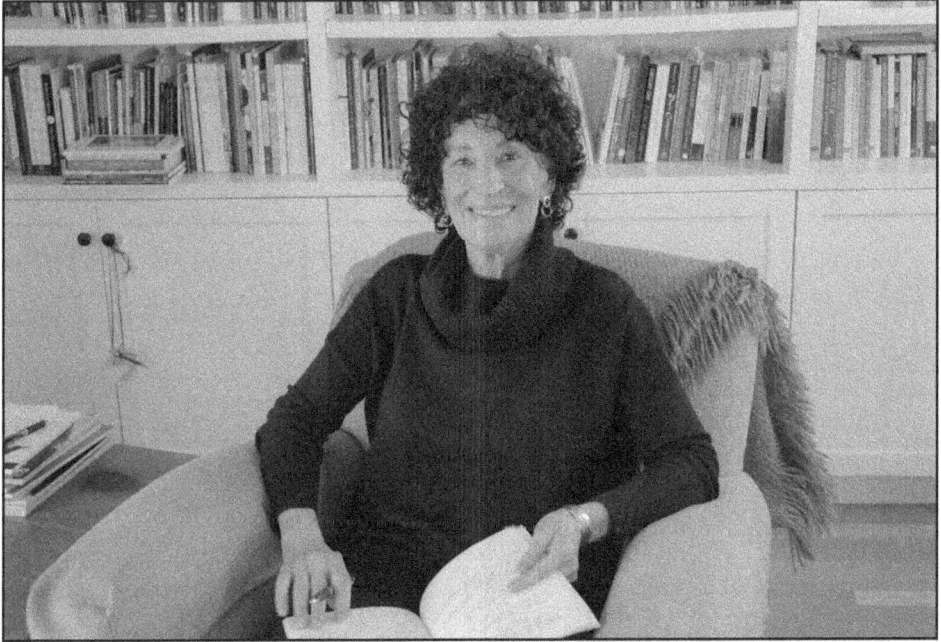

Q: Barbara, tell us about your teaching activities

A: I've been a teacher all my adult life, dramatics the first twenty years out of college, then creative writing. What lights me up is seeing students gain confidence in the process of learning as their work becomes more powerful—watching them honor it, their excitement.

Once I decided to concentrate on writing, and was accepted in the master's program at Vermont College of Fine Arts, I was blessed before graduating in 1998 with some amazingly effective teachers, Mark Cox, Clare Rossini, David Wojahn to name three. They pushed me to make uncomfortable discoveries about my work, identified strengths and weaknesses that I hadn't seen. So many generous human beings whom I try to emulate, living and breathing the writing life.

Though I've been leading poetry groups for eighteen years, during the last few I've held themed workshops in my home for six to eight students. We gather in the morning from ten to twelve around the dining-room table, once a week for six to eight weeks. Each week I pass out copies of published work, we discuss craft, and I give a homework assignment.

In the love and loss workshop, we explore life's gifts and deletions through known poems dealing with ecstasy, transience, absence, and through the students' own efforts. Recently for their homework poem I suggested they ask a dead person they'd been close to for advice on how best to live their lives. Sometimes I ask students to address mundane questions like, "Is it too icy to walk the dog this early?"

For a recent epistolary workshop, we studied the letters of the Chinese poet Yu Xuanji. She wrote to neighbors and friends in the ninth century AD—a Daoist nun executed at age twenty-eight for being too outspoken. Every letter was a poem of five stanzas, three short lines each stanza, like a gathering of haiku. Her letters are called 'matched poems' because she expected answers. For homework I asked each student to email another student in Yu Xuanji's style, and to send a response to an email received. My students dove into this; we all love to send and get letters. The women brought their two emails to the table a week later to read aloud and hear encouraging critique from others and from me.

A nurse practitioner who'd signed up leaned into every word I shared. She's since become a sophisticated poet whose work appears in journals. She's discovered other teachers whose expertise differs from mine, put together her own writing group, and completed a book-length manuscript that's found a publisher. I asked what motivated her. She said for a long time she'd felt compelled to make something with her hands, as a legacy for her children.

Another workshop I facilitate is Just Write! It's geared to women midway into a project—prose, poetry, or memoir—who need support, as well as for women wanting to start the juices flowing. I bring samples of published work that we read aloud. In our two hours together, I'll give prompts to jump-start a couple of rounds of associative writing, which encourages students not to lift their pens, to tap into their unconscious, see where the mind wanders. After we read from Rebecca Solnit's memoir, *The Faraway Nearby*, in which apricots become an ongoing image, I asked students to find an image from their own lives that haunts them, and write out several memories incorporating it.

Many women sign up for Just Write! year after year, to build trust and generate riskier material. A former marketing writer has been with us for four years. I've seen her move from a stilted, hesitant voice to a fluent treatment of a traumatic past. She's on fire, having discovered the thread for a memoir which she says she wouldn't have attempted without the group's support. When I'm not teaching, the group meets at a member's house every other week, socializing and sharing drafts of current work. They call their sessions Cocktails and Carrots.

Since 2011 I've taught a weekly class at the community college from six to eight p.m. called Women Write Their Lives. Those who have day jobs can attend, and it costs half as much as my private workshops. I love this class because of the variety of students. This fall it included a retired kindergarten teacher, a veterinary acupuncturist, a former college dean, the librarian at IAIA (Institute of American Indian Arts), a college junior, and a recently unemployed Comcast technician. The class focuses on well-known writers such as Virginia Woolf and Adrienne Rich to inspire students to find their own voice. We also hold conversations about the marginalizing of women in our culture and the arts.

Over six weeks, the former Comcast employee became increasingly passionate about her in-class writing. She shared that she'd caught her husband reading her journal, so hid it in her glove compartment. She said the class gave her courage to remove it from the car and tell her husband to lay hands off. He complied. Triumph!

I like to give prompts that stir things up. As one class's final exercise, I asked each student to write about her first sexual encounter. A woman, outraged, phoned to complain that the request was inappropriate. Another said, "I applaud you. This is the kind of risk-taking we signed up to do."

I also teach in the Wingspan Poetry Project at the Esperanza Shelter for Battered Families. Once a week women and children gather in the shelter's living room for an hour or so. Two other volunteers and I trade off. We bring each participant a blank journal and a pen. I remember one exclaiming, "I haven't been given a gift for years!" We read aloud confessional work by poets like Rita Dove, Pablo Neruda, Lucille Clifton, and Raymond Carver. Inevitably the talk morphs into what most touches attendees. They all then do associative writing for fifteen minutes.

A nine-year-old boy with shaggy brown hair and brown eyes, eager and confident, penned a four-page poem about an imagined video game. The work started as a hero's journey through the stages of hell, ending in a love/hate relationship with his father. After an hour I asked, "Are you done?"

"I'm done," he sighed. "I'm tired."

In 2015 I taught a workshop at Ghost Ranch in Abiquiu, northwest of Santa Fe, for A Room Of Her Own Foundation, a nonprofit that supports women writers through thousand-dollar prizes given twice a year for fiction, nonfiction, and poetry. Every other year the Foundation awards the fifty-thousand-dollar Gift of Freedom prize. For a hundred writers chosen from around the world, the organization also holds a biennial retreat—workshops, panels, and readings.

I called my workshop Excavating Home: Embracing the Domestic Image. In it, fifteen women, ages twenty to seventy, Anglo, African-American, Puerto Rican, and Asian-American stretched their imaginations. I asked them to walk in memory through their childhood homes, discover an object—a skillet, an overflowing ashtray, ice skates, a throw rug, whatever seemed to radiate energy—and write about it. My roommate at Ghost Ranch was blonde, witty, and athletic. The tears ran down her face as she read to the group memories evoked by the brush her mother had used to tame her hair and that of her sisters.

You may be wondering why I concentrate on teaching women. It's because their voices continue to have less clout than those of their male counterparts. In most literary publications, less than ten percent of the writing is by women. I'm becoming more and more of a feminist.

Q: What life experiences have contributed to your enthusiasm for teaching?

A: My dad was my original motivator. An Army doctor in the Philippines in World War II, he was five foot nine with wavy, auburn hair and horn-rimmed glasses. Later, seeing patients in private practice, he always wore a bow tie. He died of prostate cancer at age seventy-two. Listening was key to building relationships, he used to say, and that a good conversation was the best medicine. A man of great compassion, he elicited stories from everyone, even my macrobiotic, hippie friends. Our house was bursting with books. Although Mother and Dad read to me, Dad also made up fables, and wrote poems and short stories. He was completing a novel when he died.

My seventh-grade teacher, Mr. Oakes, was another inspiration. He asked us to write poems and essays for homework, and had us read the greats, Mark Twain, Edith Wharton, Shakespeare. But the writer who excited me most was Robert Frost. I grew up in Pittsfield, Massachusetts, the same kind of country as his Vermont meadows and woods. I could see his birches and pastures, the stone walls. My seventh-grade year I wrote and memorized an essay about an imaginary friendship with Frost, and recited it in an oratory contest.

On a cold, January night, my parents drove me to Williams College, half an hour from home, to hear Frost read. It was 1963, the year when he died at age eighty-nine. I remember being awed by that dimly lit, walnut-paneled room, listening to him bring poems I loved to life. I understood for the first time that a flesh-and-blood human being is behind any language on the page.

After editing *Rumor*, my high school's literary magazine, I went to

Syracuse University, intending to major in journalism. But since I couldn't take the pertinent courses until my junior year, I focused on my second choice for a major, theater—becoming so enamored with directing that I never did take a journalism class. Nor, after one class in poetry, did I ever take another creative writing class. The professor covered my efforts in red marks, dismissing my hard work.

Leaving Syracuse before my senior year, I worked as a director and stage manager in New York City. This morphed into teaching creative dramatics to children—using improvisation to develop scenes and fables, to kick-start the kids into developing and performing their own stories. What I loved about this is what I love about teaching writing now, creating community and trust through shared exercises. And how each student comes to believe in her innate power.

Q: Any current role models who inspire you?

A: Carole Maso is an avant-garde writer who, at this time, teaches at Brown University. In a workshop at the Millay Colony in New York, she encouraged us to dive deeply into memory and blend it with the present. She ignores trends, melds poetry and surrealism into wildly original fiction.

The poet Marie Howe is also a role model, a regal presence in flowing skirts and tunics. I've done two weeklong workshops with her at the Mabel Dodge Luhan House in Taos, and spent three weeks in a residency at Atlantic Center for the Arts in New Smyrna Beach, Florida. She, too, refuses to bow to the current literary scene. Once she picked up a fifteen-hundred-page *Norton Anthology of Poetry* and threw it across the room, saying, "We don't need this, we'll start fresh." She's more interested in creating a few beautifully wrought books than in saturating the market with them. Of her three books, *The Good Thief* remains my favorite. It features domestic poems that are fierce and honest.

Q: How do you arrange the rest of your life to let you do this good work?

A: I write almost every day, sometimes for an hour, sometimes four. Four hours is a gift; it energizes my day. And almost every night I read in bed, right now Kimberly Johnson's poetry collection, *a metaphorical god*; Elizabeth Gilbert's novel, *The Signature of All Things*; and Patti Smith's memoir, *M Train*.

Nine writers, ages forty-eight to seventy-two, three fiction writers and six poets mostly in California, are essential to my life. We call ourselves The Flamingos, birds famous for flamboyance and synchronized dance. We met at A Room Of Her Own retreat at Ghost Ranch, and reconvene every spring for a week at Sea Ranch, north of San Francisco. In between, we communicate by email and phone, trade writing with each other, and ask for feedback.

I have five dear friends in Santa Fe and one in Albuquerque whom I think of as sisters. A couple of them are writers. And there are many other women, including some of my students, I might write or share coffee with.

Most mornings I go for a three-mile, forty-minute walk, every day the same route. Not only does it serve to keep me in the moment, but breathing fresh air helps me think about my work and the glories of the natural world.

Rick, my husband, held a nine-to-five job up until his retirement. He was the worker bee who allowed me to pursue my passion as a teacher and writer.

Q: What effect does religious or spiritual practice have on your teaching and writing?

A: Buddhist authors like Pema Chodron, Sharon Salzburg, and Thich Nat Hanh, plus the Catholic priest Thomas Merton, spur me to demonstrate gratitude and loving kindness, to build mindful relationships with everyone I meet, even the shoppers lined up at Trader Joe's. I read and reread the poet Charles Wright for solace, the way others might go to the *New Testament*.

After my walk but before starting to write, I look out the living room window and list what I'm grateful for—this morning the mist over Sun Mountain, the towhee puffing its feathers on the deck's railing, the piñons gleaming with ice. I sit with my journal in half-dream for half an hour, practicing slow breathing.

All this helps create, when I'm teaching, what a student once described as "a pastoral space where we can write anxiety-free." That space allows them, I believe, to reach deeper into the unconscious than they would be able to do otherwise.

Q: What doubts and disappointments do you deal with in your work?

A: Longtime students have said, "You're so empowered in your teaching, why don't you have the same confidence as a writer?" It's true, I'm full of doubt. I don't submit my work widely because I have such high expectations of myself.

In my poem dealing with killings in a Nigerian mall, for instance, I want readers to feel enraged. In my poem about how hard marriage is, I want to unleash laughter and tears. I want to reveal the most difficult truths: my Jewish mother's anti-Semitism; facing my own sagging body; women embracing their wildness, their lust for life; the brutal, cultural pressures that my two daughters and all women feel to look and dress and act a certain way.

Disappointments as a teacher? The students who have dropped out of my classes because they found the critiques too harsh. They were unprepared to hear the truth, that making a work of art requires revision and craft. They saw the writing of poetry simply as an outpouring of emotion.

I recall a man in his early eighties bringing a full-length manuscript—single-spaced, hardly any margins—to a six-week poetry class at the community college, expecting the others and me to spend all our time responding to his masterpiece. Tall, lean, and distinguished-looking, he sought praise, not honest feedback. What could we offer him? Nothing. Though he stayed and did the exercises, he did not have, as the Buddhists put it, a beginner's mind.

In my memoir classes, students have left because they felt uncomfortable reading their homework aloud, convinced others in the class were far more talented. It takes enormous courage to enter and share the intimacies of our lives.

Q: How about a couple more examples of your successes?

A: I'm thinking about a woman in my Just Write! workshop—sixtyish, traveled the world, beautifully made-up, hair streaked blonde—struggling with a memoir about her life in the sixties as a photographer and publicist for entertainers like Wavy Gravy and rock bands like Crosby, Stills, Nash, and Young. At first her writing meandered, was mostly just snippets, but after half a dozen drafts, the sequencing flowed. Thanks to her perseverance in class, and the help of an independent critique group she formed, the memoir was of high enough quality to start submitting for publication.

Then there were the three women who returned for five years to eight-week poetry workshops I ran in the winter, spring, and fall. They put together an anthology called *Braided Voices* that sold for ten dollars in local bookstores, following a packed launch at the Santa Fe Woman's Club. One wrote humorous, story-telling poems about New Mexico. Another wrote surreal poems about her Hawaiian heritage. The third wrote from her perspective as a nurse and about her brother's schizophrenia.

Barbara Rockman's Thumbnail Bio:

Born in Pittsfield, Massachusetts, 1949. BA in Education, University Without Walls, Roger Williams College, Rhode Island, 1976. MEd., Antioch University, NH, 1978. MFA in Writing, Vermont College of Fine Arts, Vermont, 1998. Taught creative dramatics and developed arts-education curricula in California, New Mexico, Massachusetts, New Hampshire, and New York, 1972–1992. Teaches creative writing at the Santa Fe Community College and in private workshops, 1998–present. Teaches in the Wingspan Poetry Project, Esperanza Shelter for Battered Families, 2014–present. Editor, *Women Becoming Poems*, Cinnabar Press, 2002. Author, poetry chapbook, *Surrender to Storm*, Cinnabar Press, 2006. Author, poetry collection, *Sting and Nest*, Sunstone Press, 2011. Prizes: New Mexico Discovery Award, 1998; Southwest Writers Prize, 2000; *The MacGuffin* National Poet Hunt, 2001; Persimmon Tree Prize, 2009; National Press Women Book Award and New Mexico-Arizona Book Award, 2012.

To get help as a writer see national websites below:

National

> Association of Writers & Writing Programs
> www.awpwriter.org
>
> Poets & Writers
> www.pw.org
>
> Academy of American Poets
> www.poets.org
>
> National Federation of State Poetry Societies
> www.nfsps.com
>
> Poetry Society of America
> www.poetrysociety.org

A Room of Her Own Foundation
www.aroomofherownfoundation.org

VIDA: Women in Literary Arts
www.vidaweb.org

In Santa Fe

Santa Fe Community College
www.sfcc.edu

Institute of Amerian Indian Arts
www.iaia.edu

University of Art and Design
www.santafeuniversity.edu

About the Type

This book has been set in Adobe Caslon Pro.

Caslon is a group of serif typefaces designed by William Caslon I (1692–1766) in London. Caslon worked as an engraver of punches, the masters used to stamp the moulds or matrices used to cast metal type. He worked in the tradition of what is now called old-style serif letter design, that produced letters with a relatively organic structure resembling handwriting with a pen. Caslon established a tradition of designing type in London, which had not been common, and so he was influenced by the imported Dutch Baroque typefaces that were popular in England at the time.

Caslon's typefaces were popular in his lifetime and beyond, and after a brief period of eclipse in the nineteenth century remain common, particularly for setting printed body text and books. Many revivals exist, with varying faithfulness to Caslon's original design.

www.ingramcontent.com/pod-product-compliance
Lightning Source LLC
Chambersburg PA
CBHW031434270326
41930CB00007B/695